DR TOM SMITH has been writing full time since 1977, after spending six years in general practice and seven years in medical research. He writes regularly for medical journals and magazines and has a weekly column in the *Bradford Telegraph and Argus*. He also broadcasts regularly for BBC Radio Scotland. His other books for Sheldon Press include *Heart Attacks: Prevent and Survive, Living with Alzheimer's Disease* and *Coping Successfully with Prostate Cancer*.

Overcoming Common Problems Series

A full list of titles is available from Sheldon Press,
1 Marylebone Road, London NW1 4DU, and on our website at
www.sheldonpress.co.uk

Overcoming Common Problems Series

Overcoming Common Problems Series

Overcoming Common Problems

Overcoming Back Pain

Dr Tom Smith

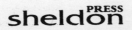

First published in Great Britain in 2003 by
Sheldon Press
1 Marylebone Road
London NW1 4DU

British Library Cataloguing-in-Publication Data

A catalogue record for this book is available from the British Library

ISBN 0–85969–883–1

1 3 5 7 9 10 8 6 4 2

Typeset by Deltatype Limited, Birkenhead, Merseyside
Printed in Great Britain by Biddles Ltd
www.biddles.co.uk

Contents

Introduction

I'm proud of my medical education. Birmingham Medical School, in the heart of the English Midlands, gave its students brilliant opportunities to study every disease of modern men and women. With a single medical school tending to a population of more than 5 million, the ratio of students to sick people was around the best in Britain. By the end of our years at the school, we felt we had encountered, and had been taught to diagnose and treat, every illness to which modern man and woman is susceptible.

For the most part, when I eventually entered general practice, this was true. With one glaring exception. Back pain. Somehow, back pain featured very little in our lectures or in our outpatient clinics. We learned a little about 'slipped discs' and sciatica and lumbago, and that was about all. Back pain was something that we could do little about, except wait until it got better. It would do that, said our lecturers, in time, provided the person with it rested. Truly, there were no people who deserved more the title of 'patients'. They had to be patient, because all they could do was wait.

However, when I got to my first practice – sole doctor, and dispenser, in a small town in a rural area in the west of Scotland – I soon found that this view of back-pain management was wholly inadequate. Active farmers, fishermen, forestry workers and road workers can't afford to wait until they are better. So I gained a reputation for referring anyone with back pain to the orthopaedic department of our local hospital. I reasoned that the consultants there would know much more than me about it, and could solve my patients' problems faster and more efficiently.

Not so. My patients, male or female, invariably returned home encased in surgical corsets, and it soon became clear to me that this wasn't the answer. All that seemed to have happened was that their backs were now stiff as well as painful. And when they finally took off the corsets, they were weak, too. The medical team was making them worse rather than better. We were failing our patients.

Happily, a chance conversation at a local medical meeting changed all that. Dr Hugh Baird, a neighbouring doctor, had trained at St Thomas's Hospital, in London. There he had come under the influence of James Cyriax, at that time the only doctor at any British medical school who carried the title of Professor of Orthopaedic Medicine. Dr Baird lent me two books by Professor Cyriax on the management of back pain. I read them, tried out his advice, and was from then on a devotee. Patients actually lost their pain, with some even walking out of my surgery free of pain for the first time in weeks. Of course, I didn't have this success every time. There were plenty of people to whom Cyriax's methods did not apply. But the success rate in reducing and curing pain was far higher than with corsets or painkillers, and at last I had practical and useful advice to offer everyone with a back problem.

James Cyriax was an orthodox physician, a distinguished academic accepted by his university-based peers, who was dedicated to restoring the idea of 'manipulative medicine' as an acceptable way to treat all sorts of muscular and skeletal pain. He was not a chiropractor or an osteopath. He wanted orthodox doctors to learn the skills of manipulation as just one part of the management of painful backs. According to him, crucial to making decisions on the treatment of back pain was the need for detailed knowledge of the structure (anatomy) and the function (physiology) of the back, and of all the problems with internal organs that might also cause back pain. Cyriax wanted to make sure that people who treat back pain have such knowledge, and he believed that only medical training gave them that knowledge.

My own view on osteopathy and chiropractic is more tolerant, but I have no training in either of them. So if you are inclined to turn to one of these branches of alternative medicine for your treatment, you should read one of the many books on them. But please dip into this one, too. In principle, it has its beginnings in Cyriax's method. However, his heyday was more than forty years ago, and knowledge of backs – and what can go wrong with them – has advanced a great deal since then.

One man in particular has led these advances. He is Gordon Waddell, Professor of Orthopaedic Surgery at the University of Glasgow and Visiting Professor at the Rheumatology Department of the University of Manchester. For many years he ran a 'Problem Back Clinic' that was famous among Scots doctors. He has received many awards for his work on back pain. He has built much-needed bridges between orthodox medicine and osteopathy, being Associate Professor of Clinical Research at the British School of Osteopathy.

INTRODUCTION

Most important for doctors interested in helping people with back pain, he wrote the 'bible' of back pain for doctors – *The Back Pain Revolution* (Waddell, 1998).

The Back Pain Revolution was written to educate doctors, and I have used its advice on many occasions to help my patients. This book is for people with back pain and for those who care for them. Necessarily, because Professor Waddell's knowledge and research has been so comprehensive, virtually all of the chapters on diagnosis and treatment of back pain have been based on his work. This is why I have dedicated my book to him. He has changed my management of back pain: I hope readers of this book will benefit just as much as my patients have.

1

Our backs and why they hurt

The back is a fairly simple structure. It is a column of interconnecting bones, the spine, held together and kept firmly in place by very strong ligaments and muscles running alongside it, and 'fixing' the spine in place relative to other structures such as the ribs, the pelvis and the front of the abdomen. Most back pain arises because the muscles have been disturbed in some way, perhaps by a simple sprain. Lifting a weight while twisting the torso is a perfect way, for example, to initiate this disturbance. We put too much strain on a particular muscle and it tears. That is followed by deep-seated bruising at the site of the muscle tear, which leads not only to pain, but also to cramp in the affected muscle. The normal way to treat cramp is to stretch the muscle. If you get cramp in a calf muscle, you pull up the foot. Get cramp in the sole of the foot, and you pull out the corresponding toe. But get sudden pain in the lower back, and we hunch up – rather than stretch – and so allow the cramp to continue. From then on we are sunk: the back muscle takes longer to recover, and the pain remains.

Sounds simple? Amazingly, for the amount of time that is spent on pain in the back, it is almost always that simple. The main problem is, in trying to ease the pain, that we often make it worse. We turn a short-term episode of back pain ('acute' backache) into a long-term one ('chronic' back pain). Sadly, there are many ways of making back pain worse, which is why there are so many people whose livelihood depends on curing it. The fact that we have treatments as widely diverse as osteopathy, chiropractic, physiotherapy, acupuncture and homoeopathy, as well as orthodox medicine and surgery, suggests that we aren't getting it right.

So how should we approach the problem of back pain? For orthodox doctors like myself, the standard way is to follow the tried and tested way by which we approach any illness. We listen to the patient's symptoms, examine them, formulate a provisional diagnosis, and perhaps add a test or two to confirm (or not, as the case might be) our initial suspicions. Having made the diagnosis, we can then make the decision on how to treat.

This system works perfectly for diseases such as asthma, or

kidney infections, or a heart attack, or diabetes. It isn't so clear-cut, though, for the causes and treatment of back pain. The main difficulty with back pain is that even experts such as Professor Waddell only find a definite disease as the cause of the pain in about one person in seven. What we can do is to rule out serious disease as the cause of the pain in the other six. We can reassure them that they don't have cancer or any other life-threatening illness. That is the good news. But the bad news is that we can't say, for certain, what they do have.

What we can offer to people with back pain is the 'diagnostic triage' developed by Professor Waddell. 'Triage' is a medical buzz-word coined around the 1980s to describe the system by which doctors and other staff in Accident and Emergency departments dealt with their new patients. It lays down the steps by which they come to conclusions and start treatment. First used for dealing with serious accidents and medical emergencies such as heart attacks and strokes, the word triage is just as applicable to back pain.

The Waddell system of triage for back pain is simplicity itself. It divides back pain into 'simple backache', 'nerve root pain' and 'possible serious spinal disease'. Most readers of this book have the first. Fewer than one person in twenty with back pain has the second. A very small minority, fewer than one in a hundred, according to Professor Waddell, have the third. The next few paragraphs will allow you to place yourself in one of these categories:

Simple backache

Simple backache arises out of the blue. It may follow a particular activity, like digging or lifting, or reaching out a little too far for something. Or twisting the lower back in an awkward way. But it can just as easily start quite spontaneously, the person being unable to remember anything that might have brought it on. Although classified as simple, it can be very painful, so that the intensity of the pain gives no clue to its type or its cause. Fundamentally it is a muscle problem, so it is much more likely to occur in people who are relatively active and relatively young – say, an adult up to the age of 50. It can spread into either buttock or thigh, is made worse or comes on with physical activity, and varies in intensity over each 24 hours. People with simple backache are otherwise well, with no other debilitating illness or problems that point to nerve damage or spinal bony problems. Most cases of what is popularly called lumbago are forms of simple backache.

Nerve root pain

The nerve root pain with which most people are familiar is sciatica. This is a pain from the middle of a buttock down the back of the thigh to the knee, and sometimes into the calf and the top of the foot. The pain in the back is less intense than the pain in the leg. As the title suggests, this pain comes from pressure on the 'nerve root', precisely at the site where the sciatic nerve carrying sensation from the leg passes through an opening between two vertebrae in the back on its way into the spinal cord.

To understand why this may happen you need to know something about the spinal vertebrae. We have five vertebrae in the back. They are the largest vertebrae in the spinal column, because they have to bear the body's weight. Between these vertebrae are discs of cartilage, not unlike ice hockey pucks, that act as shock absorbers, so that the bones do not 'crunch' one against the other when we are in the upright position. Alongside the discs there are spaces between the vertebrae through which the nerves must pass into and from the spinal cord. The nerves entering the cord are those that carry sensation (touch, pain, the recognition of heat and cold, a sense of position in space, and vibration sense) from the body to the brain. The nerves exiting the cord are the ones that control muscle activity. Anatomists are logical, so these nerves are called the sensory and motor nerves. The sensory nerves enter through the channels at the back of the spine and the motor nerves emerge from the front of the spine.

Anything that may cause the nerves not to function correctly, such as a bulging disc, or a collapsed vertebra leading to narrowing of the nerve-bearing channels, can lead therefore to a mixture of symptoms. You may have pain on its own, but you may also experience pins and needles, lose the ability to feel hot and cold in the area affected, and even find it difficult to know where your feet are in space. If the bulge is a little further forward, your main problem may be weakness as the motor nerve is affected.

There are five lumbar vertebrae, and the nerves emerging and entering between each pair of vertebrae have different areas of distribution. Nerve roots higher in the column will affect the back and groin: as you go down the 'ladder' the nerves supply the groin and upper inner thigh, the buttock and leg down to the knee, and then the shin and foot accordingly. It is not necessary to go into the anatomy in detail here: it is enough to accept that a pinpoint description of exactly where you feel pain, and of exactly which muscles are weak, will tell your doctor precisely where in the spine the nerve root is being compressed.

In general, if nerve root pressure is the cause of backache, the pain is worse in the leg than in the back, it usually affects only one side, and it is often accompanied (paradoxically) by numbness and/or pins and needles in the same area as the pain. If you have this sort of pain, it is made worse if, when you lie on your back, someone lifts up your leg, with the knee straight. This 'straight leg lifting test' has been a classical test for sciatica for hundreds of years. The problem is that many people with backache know about it – and that can be a complication in making the diagnosis of true nerve root pain. We will return to this later in the book.

Serious spinal disease

Before we start on the signs of serious back pain, do remember that it accounts for less than 1 per cent of all cases of back pain seen by doctors. So be reassured that it is rare, and that it isn't diagnosed without making certain that there are less serious causes for the pain. The most serious back pain of all is caused by tumours (cancers) of the spine, which have either arisen there as primary disease or have spread there from other organs (secondary cancer or 'metastases'). Other back pains classified as 'serious' are caused by infections in the bones of the spine or in the tissues in and around the spinal cord, or by 'inflammatory' diseases such as ankylosing spondylitis, about which more later.

In trying to sort out the less serious from the more serious causes of back pain, Professor Waddell has listed the 'red flag' problems that point to serious spinal disease. They include pain:

- starting before the person is 20 or after the age of 55;
- after a serious accident, such as a fall from a height, or a traffic accident;

- that is always there regardless of position, exercise, a particular movement or rest;
- in the back of the chest rather than in the lower back;
- in a person with a history of previous cancer in, say, the breast or prostate;
- in someone taking long-term cortisone-like drugs by mouth;
- in a person who is abusing illegal drugs;
- in someone with HIV/AIDS;
- that accompanies weight loss in a person who feels generally unwell;
- with severe stiffness of the back preventing bending forwards;
- with signs that nerves to the limbs or other regions are also affected;
- that includes an obvious deformity of the back, such as a sideways bend.

Other symptoms that strongly suggest a serious spinal problem include difficulty in passing urine and/or the ability to control opening of the bowels, loss of feeling around the anus, the perineum (the area between the anus and the genitals), and/or the genitals. Any weakness of the muscles of the back or legs, and loss of the ability to feel touch and pinprick in the lower back or limbs, is also a pointer to serious back disease.

'Inflammatory' diseases of the spine have their own particular set of symptoms, which together make the diagnosis fairly obvious. People who develop such problems usually start to feel something is wrong before they reach their forties. Often the first symptom is stiff muscles when they wake each morning. They become less flexible, so that their ability to move their spines in any direction is much more restricted than before. Along with their back pain, they often have stiff swollen wrist and finger joints, and perhaps in joints such as the ankles, toes, elbows and knees. Along with these multiple joint symptoms come eye inflammation ('iritis'), skin problems such as psoriasis and other less well-recognized rashes, bowel upsets such as colitis, and even urinary discharges that turn out not to be infectious when samples are sent to the lab for culture. Often there are, or have been, close relatives with a similar problem.

Faced with all these symptoms, your doctor will take a simple blood test to confirm or rule out inflammation as a cause of the pain. This is an 'erythrocyte sedimentation rate', or ESR. It is the rate at which, in a column of blood taken from a vein, the red cells separate downwards from the plasma in which they float. The faster they settle, the more likely there is to be an inflammatory process going on in the body. A normal blood sample will show an ESR under 10 centimetres per hour. In people with inflammatory disease, it can be many times that, and certainly above 25 centimetres per hour. If your ESR is high, then you will have further blood tests to confirm the diagnosis, and perhaps identify the type of inflammation that you have. On that will depend the type of medical treatment you need.

Ankylosing spondylitis is an inflammation of the joints between the vertebrae, which over many years causes 'bridges' of rigid bone to form between them. The spine ends up so stiff that the sufferer loses all flexibility. On X-rays, the spinal column comes to look like a length of bamboo, so that the appearance is called 'bamboo spine'. In the past, early ankylosing spondylitis was treated with X-rays to stop the formation of the bony bridges across the joints, but when tumours arose years later in the irradiated areas, the practice was stopped. Now people with this illness are asked to do regular exercises to keep the spine flexible, and take anti-arthritic drugs to keep the stiffening process at bay. It is an inherited condition, mostly started in the late teens, and gradually worsens over many years. With energetic treatment and enthusiastic exercise, most sufferers nowadays avoid the worst of the stiffening and immobility. Ankylosing spondylitis need not shorten life. In fact, such treatment is a shining example of how regular exercise can defeat a back condition.

2

Pinpointing the cause

So here you are in the doctor's room, with your complaint of back pain. The absolute first step that your doctor will take is to find out whether the pain is really coming from a problem in your back – that is, the muscles, joints or bones that make up the structures in the back. That isn't as obvious or clear-cut as it sounds. Pain in the back may arise from an illness affecting other organs, but that the brain interprets as coming from the back. The pain may actually be coming from a problem in an internal organ, such as the kidneys, the gallbladder, the pancreas, the stomach or bowel. In women it may arise from the ovaries or womb, and in men from the prostate gland. There may be problems in the hip joints. The pain may even be a problem of the circulation, so that the blood flow through narrowed arteries to an area of the back may be poor. With exertion, this blood flow may become too little to sustain an adequate oxygen supply to the back muscles or spine, and this can give rise to a pain that comes on with exercise, and dies away when you rest.

I have very good reason to remember that form of back pain. As a young GP, I saw an elderly woman with pain in the middle of her back that came on when she undertook gentle exercise. At first I thought it was a form of angina, with the pain coming from her heart, but her electrocardiogram (ECG) was normal. However, she did have diabetes, and very poor circulation in her feet, a common complication of long-standing diabetes. I came to the conclusion that the arteries supplying blood to the middle region of her spine were as narrow as those to her feet, and that her pain was a form of 'angina' affecting her spinal cord.

I arranged for her to be seen by a vascular specialist, with a view to possible surgery, or at least appropriate medical treatment, and advised her to rest as much as she could until she saw him. Unfortunately, she was needed by her employers (she was a housekeeper), and rather than allow her to rest, they took her to a man who in those days was described as a 'bone setter'. Tragically, he manipulated her back, and she became permanently paralysed from the waist down. The manipulation had finally blocked off her ailing artery, and the area of spinal cord that it had supplied with blood died off. The technical term for this is an 'infarct', and there is no possibility of recovery from it.

So before anyone takes the decision to manipulate or stretch the spine, they must make sure that they will not do harm. They can only do that if they rule out all possible causes of the pain that might not respond, or might respond badly, to such treatment. So the first rule for anyone treating back pain is to take a thorough history of the pain and to perform a thorough physical examination. If the pain is caused by disease of an internal organ, there are usually other symptoms that point to this.

For example, pain radiating to the back from a diseased gallbladder is made worse after eating fatty foods. People with gallbladder problems are often tender just under the margin of the ribs in the front of the abdomen, to the right of the midline. A swelling liver, perhaps due to hepatitis or other liver disease, may start with the same symptoms. Back pain that is really indigestion, due to stomach ulcers or an inflamed stomach, is often linked to pain in the front of the abdomen, above the navel, in what doctors call the epigastrium. Back pain caused by pancreas problems is usually a constant dull boring ache, also in the epigastrium. Back pain linked to kidney trouble centres upon the angle between the ribs and the spine on either side. It may radiate down and around the front of the abdomen, into the groin and, in men, into one testicle.

In women, back pain arising from troubles in the uterus and cervix is usually lower down the back, and feels vaguely in the middle of the back, on either side. In younger women who are still menstruating, it is usually worse in the latter half of the menstrual cycle. Causes can vary from fibroids in the uterus (a form of benign overgrowth of the uterine muscle), to chronic infections in the cervix and in the tubes leading from the ovaries to the uterus. Cystic ovaries can also cause back pain, on one side or the other.

In older women, past their menopause, back pain due to womb problems is more likely to be associated with prolapse, in which the muscle support within the pelvis that keeps the womb, bladder and/ or bowel in place has been lost. That allows any or all of these organs to fall downwards into the vagina, and leads to a dragging pain in the back.

In men over 50 who start to have back pain, the prostate gland comes under suspicion. An enlarging prostate gland may well cause pain in the back. And if it is a malignant enlargement, there may be secondary spread to the bones of the pelvis and spine, which can cause severe back pain. In fact, back pain may be the first and only indication that a man has prostate cancer.

So if you have started to have back pain, do not be surprised if your doctor asks you to undergo a full examination of the abdomen, as well as the back. Tenderness in the upper abdomen may well point to stomach, gallbladder or pancreatic problems. Tenderness on the left side of the front of the abdomen may mean diverticular disease of the large bowel (the colon). Tenderness in the angles between the ribs and spine may indicate kidney problems. And tenderness in the centre of the lowest part of the abdomen, just above the pelvic bone (the pubis), could mean a chronic bladder problem.

After this examination, you may then be asked to consent to an 'internal'. If your story is appropriate and the abdominal examination suggests possible disease in the pelvis (ovary, womb and cervix in a woman, the prostate gland in a man), you will need a rectal and/ or vaginal examination. Such procedures may seem embarrassing and uncomfortable, but they are essential, in some cases, in finding out the facts. Not everyone with backache needs an internal examination, but if your doctor asks for one, it is advisable to consent to it.

If the doctor finds anything suspicious, you will be asked to have further tests. Blood may be taken to check on your liver and kidney function, and on your cholesterol levels, which may point to gallbladder disease. Men will almost certainly be tested for prostate-specific antigen (PSA), which will indicate whether or not there is prostate cancer, and can even give a reasonable assessment of whether and how much it has spread. For more about PSA and prostate cancer, please refer to *Coping Successfully with Prostate Cancer* (Smith, 2002).

Your doctor will also ask you to walk up and down. Pain in the back may come from a hip joint. When hips begin to degenerate, and the normal space within the joint that separates the upper part of the thigh bone (the femur) from the pelvis begins to disappear, you start to limp. With one leg now essentially shorter than the other, your back is tilted, and the muscles on one side of the back contract to even up the spine. The natural result is a sideways tilt of the spine, and a sore back as the muscles on one side do much more work than those on the other side. So although you feel the pain in the back, the area that needs treatment is the hip joint. Part of your doctor's examination, therefore, is to put your hip joint through its normal range of movement. If that is restricted, especially if there is pain when the doctor tries to do this, then the hip joint comes under suspicion as the cause of your pain.

By now you will be beginning to understand that pain that your brain interprets as coming from your back isn't actually doing so. Back pain is much more complex than it first appears. Your doctor has to go through a strict routine if there is any suspicion that the pain is more than a simple muscular backache. Once more serious problems have been ruled out, your doctor can then get on with making a diagnosis and managing the pain.

Diagnosing the type of back pain

So let us go through what should be done to sort out the different sorts of back pain.

Simple back pain

If, after you have answered a few questions and been examined, and your doctor decides that this is a simple 'mechanical' back pain – usually a muscle 'pull' or strain – then you can start the treatment. There is no need for any further investigations. How this pain should be treated is dealt with in Chapters 7 and 8. This applies even in most cases of pain down a leg, the pain usually referred to as 'sciatica'. Most cases of sciatica are simple muscle strains in the back, and not due to a 'slipped' or 'bulging' disc. In fact, sciatica is most of the time a misnomer, because it is not caused by pressure on the sciatic nerve as it enters the spine, but by muscle spasms or cramps in the back. The pain has a vague distribution, usually affecting the buttocks and thighs, often on both sides, but rarely spreading much below the knee. It is more of a dull ache than a severe, stabbing pain. This sort of pain arises from strains in ligaments, the small joints between the vertebrae, the muscles around them, or even the surface 'skin' of the bone, the 'periosteum'. It leads to cramps in the muscles around the lower spine and in the buttocks and thighs. Doctors prefer to call it 'referred pain', rather than sciatica, to show that the brain refers the site of the pain to the leg, when it is actually in the muscles of the lower back. The next chapter, on the way we feel pain, explains this in more detail.

Nerve root pain

However, if your doctor suspects that your pain is caused by something more than a back muscle strain or cramp, you will need a more detailed 'work-up'. As mentioned in the last chapter, around 5 per cent of all back pains – only around one in twenty – are diagnosed as being 'nerve root' pains. That is, they arise directly from pressure on a nerve as it enters the gap between two vertebrae on its way into the spinal cord. The vast majority of such nerve root pains (according to Professor Waddell's research) involve the space between the fourth and fifth lumbar (back) vertebrae and the space between the fifth vertebra and the top of the pelvic bone – the sacrum.

The pain that such nerve root pressures cause is very specific, and is precisely in the distribution of the corresponding nerves (the area of skin and muscles in which each nerve acts). For the sciatic nerve, it passes down the back of the thigh on one side, running along the outside surface of the lower leg and into the top and outside margin of the foot. Such pressure on a nerve doesn't simply give pain. These nerves carry other sensations as well as that of pain, so that when pressure is put upon them they disturb the nerve function in several ways. That is why with nerve root pain you may find that a patch of skin in the thigh or lower leg may be completely numb, so that you don't feel a pin prick, or can't tell the difference between the blunt and sharp ends of a needle when they are pressed against the skin. It also explains why you may feel 'pins and needles' in the feet and legs, or why you can't tell the difference between hot and cold test tubes when applied to the skin. You may not know exactly where your feet are when you are walking, because the 'position sense' nerves may have been damaged, along with the others.

Along with these symptoms come more subtle signs that the nerve has been damaged. There may be weakness in the ankle, foot and toes that you may not have noticed, but which the doctor can pick up with a meticulous examination, usually by comparing the relative strengths of the muscles in the two legs. Your ankle jerk reflex (the strength of the response of the foot when your Achilles tendon is struck with a rubber hammer) may be much less than normal.

So the examination of the leg is vital to differentiating between a simple back pain and damage to a nerve in the back causing root pain. It can't be too strongly stressed that a pain down a leg is not evidence of a disc problem, causing pressure on a nerve, without other corroborating evidence that can be produced from a careful history and examination. Making that differentiation is very important, because it makes a big difference to how the pain will be treated and managed.

More serious spinal disease

If your doctor suspects that you have more serious spinal disease than a simple muscular problem or nerve root pressure, then you will be asked to undergo further tests. The one that most people think of first is an X-ray of the back. In fact the first question asked by many people with back pain is 'Shouldn't I have an X-ray?' It is never as simple as that. First of all, X-rays only show problems with bones and perhaps the spaces between them. They do not show problems with muscles and tendons, or even with discs, so that they add absolutely nothing to the doctor's knowledge of a simple or nerve root-induced pain. And even if they do show some degeneration of the spinal vertebrae, this is a feature of most people who have no back pain. Nor will a 'normal' back X-ray rule out the presence of disease in the bones, such as early secondary deposits ('metastases') of cancer from the prostate or breast, both of which are causes of back pain in people with serious spinal disease. Metastases may be there (and cause pain) for many months before they have done enough damage to the bones to show up in a straight X-ray.

So do not be surprised or disappointed if your doctor isn't happy to agree to your request for an X-ray. It will hardly ever show the cause of your pain, and the extra exposure to X-rays is an added risk. I quote Professor Waddell: 'A standard set of three lumbosacral [back] X-rays gives 120 times the radiation dose of a chest X-ray.' Unless there is a very good reason for performing an X-ray on the back, the drawbacks will exceed the benefits.

What about more sophisticated techniques, such as computerized tomography (CAT) and magnetic resonance imaging (MRI) scans? They show the spine and its surrounding tissues in amazing detail, and will spot metastases and indicate exactly where nerve roots are compressed. But they are only for use once these diagnoses have been made from other tests. Surgeons can then rely upon them to plan their operations to relieve pressure exactly. Cancer specialists use them to pinpoint their attack (with radiation treatment or cancer-attacking drugs), then repeat them to follow up their response. But CAT and MRI scans are not used in the initial diagnostic scheme, when what is needed is to place the patient in one of the three categories of 'simple', 'nerve root' or 'serious'. It would also be impossible to use them in every case of backache. There just aren't enough machines and operators to cope with such a demand, and it would be a waste of these valuable resources, which are needed for many other diseases, where their use is much more critical to the diagnosis. In any case, what would you do with a person who has no nerve root symptoms, but whose CAT scan showed a bulging disc? Surgeons cannot decide to operate on a CAT scan result alone. The person's pain may well be nothing to do with the disc, and will still be there when they recover from a major operation. No operation is without risk, and there is no point in performing one if the chances of a good outcome are slim.

In the past this was not a rare event, and it gave spinal surgery a bad name. Spinal surgeons are very aware of these 'false positive' cases, and will not operate unless there is definite evidence, along the lines of the paragraph above, that real disease of the spine, or the nerves emerging from it, is causing the pain. Today's surgeons will always try to match the findings from their examinations and tests with the patient's actual complaints, and come to a definite diagnostic conclusion, before considering whether or not to operate, and what form the operation will take. Having one or more of the 'red flag' problems listed on pages 4–5, Chapter 1, will have much more influence, initially, on what is to be done than X-rays and scans.

3
Pain is just part of the problem

Be warned before you read this chapter, because it may annoy you. Presumably you are reading this book because you have, or someone close to you has, back pain. You may be so damaged by it that you can't work or pursue a normal life. You may have lost your job; the pain may even have broken up your marriage, because of all the frustrations that disability due to 'a bad back' can bring. Your pain is, to you, the one thing that has ruined your life.

But is that really so? If you were told that there are people in many countries who have back pain at least as bad as yours, but have to go on living and working with it because they have no alternative, how would you feel? Do you feel the anger starting to rise within you? If so, you are not alone. One of the problems of having back pain in our developed society is that there is little sympathy for the back-pain sufferer. You may even have been faced with the accusation that you are using your pain to avoid work, or to raise sympathy, or even to avoid responsibilities that you don't wish to face.

There is some basis for these accusations, however unfair you think they are. Until around 1998, chronic back pain was one of the most common reasons for people to be signed off work. The usual treatment for back pain until then was rest. It is so easy to fake back pain, and doctors had no real means of sorting out what was real and what was, to put it kindly, 'put on'. They would be forced, sometimes against their better judgement, to sign people off work almost as long as they wished, until the pain eased. When it eased was often determined by the person's desire to go back to work, for financial, rather than health, reasons.

Amazingly, this all changed after a report in the medical press that the best way to relieve back pain was to exercise the back muscles, rather than to rest them. It was widely publicized that back pain was no longer an excuse to rest or stop work. In fact, going to work was a positive part of the treatment! I must admit, as a GP at the time, this news came as a great relief.

It was also very instructive. Because after that time, GPs like myself were able to concentrate on the people with genuinely disabling back pain. It soon became clear that it is the disability that pain brings, rather than the pain itself, that is the problem. Many people who have severe back pain because of serious disease in the spine go to work, cope well, and manage to enjoy a reasonable quality of life. Others with what is diagnosed as simple back pain (see Chapter 1 for the definition), with no serious disease showing up on CAT or MRI scans, are wholly incapacitated by their pain and never work again.

To understand why this is so, you have to know something more about the nature of pain. We used to think that pain is simply an unpleasant reaction to something that has happened to you. It was thought to be predictable, like the reaction of an experimental animal to a measured pressure gauge on a paw. The more the pressure, the more the unfortunate animal would react, and each animal would react in a similar way. But that isn't so for human pain.

It is true that we have nerves in our skin, muscles and some internal organs, like our gut, that carry electrical stimuli from injured or inflamed areas, first to the spinal cord, and then to the brain, where they are interpreted as pain. But that isn't the whole story. On the way to the brain, these pain-inducing signals can be modified by other signals from other sites, so that they are perceived as not so severe, or even more severe. This is called the 'gate' theory of pain, first described by Melzack and Wall in 1965 (Melzack and Wall, 1965, pp. 971–9). It isn't necessary to go into detail on the gate theory here, but because it helps to explain why the perception of pain differs from person to person, and why individuals respond in a variety of ways to different treatments, it is helpful to know the basic principles of the gate theory.

Melzack and Wall originally saw things in the following way:

1 A part of the body is injured or inflamed.
2 Nerve endings at the site of the injury or disease pick up the chemical changes that it has caused.
3 This 'message' is transformed by the nerve into an electrical current that travels along the nerve to the spinal cord, where the message is passed on to another nerve that relays it up the spinal cord into the brain.
4 The brain receives the message and the person becomes conscious of it as pain. We only feel the pain when it reaches the brain, which tells us its exact origin.

So where did the 'gate' come in? At each level of this long pathway from skin or muscle or gut to the brain, the message may be modified by other messages coming in from other nerves or other chemical changes. Let us take a very old example. Roman soldiers during their occupation of Britain carried stinging nettles with them. They were prone to rheumatic pains in their joints and muscles – clearly, our climate must have been as damp and cold then as it is now. I am writing this book in the summer of 2002, the worst, coldest and dampest in Britain in living memory.

When they were in pain, the Romans used to rub the nettles on the affected spots. The stinging sensation caused a different type of pain 'message' to pass along the same nerve bundles. This interfered with their rheumatic pain message, and they felt better. In effect, they used one form of pain to neutralize the other. Rubbing stinging nettles on your skin is a bit drastic, but it is the same principle as putting a hot water bottle, a cold compress, or a liniment rub on the area. The pain message is lessened because the extra stimulus to the skin interferes with it. This is called 'counter-irritation', and creams and ointments that apply heat to the skin to ease pain are classified as 'rubefacients' – meaning that they make the skin to which they are applied red.

A development on from this principle is the TENS machine. TENS stands for Transcutaneous Electrical Nerve Stimulation. It repeatedly delivers tiny electrical shocks to the skin over the area of pain. Its effect is to block out the pain signals travelling along the nerve bundle that is carrying the pain message. Many people with chronic pain find TENS a huge benefit. Sadly, it does not work for others.

These pain-modifying messages do not have to originate near the site of the pain to have their effects. One example appears to be acupuncture. We do not know precisely how acupuncture works to ease pain, but some people get relief from it, and the needles used are usually positioned in areas quite unrelated to the point of pain. It is difficult for anyone trained in human anatomy to accept the existence of the meridian lines used by acupuncturists, as they have never been shown to have any structure inside the body.

However, the needles may release a chemical 'messenger' into the bloodstream that modifies the perception of pain in the brain. Everyone by now has heard of endorphins, the morphine-like painkilling and sedative substances that arc produced by the brain as a reaction to illness or to exercise. It is claimed that acupuncture releases endorphins from the brain, and that they are the reason for its effect. I do not know of any studies that have confirmed this theory. They would be difficult to do, because the endorphin levels would have to be measured in spinal fluid before and after the acupuncture, and it is hardly ethical to subject people to what is essentially a surgical procedure with definite risks if their only complaint is simple pain.

One warning about acupuncture. Years ago, I had a very good friend in Dr Siang Liem, a Dutch doctor, of Chinese origin. We worked together in research into new drugs, so he was exceptionally knowledgeable in modern, orthodox medicine. He was also, because of his ethnic background, very well versed in acupuncture, and for years was the President of the Dutch Acupuncture Society. I asked him about the use of acupuncture in pain. He agreed that it was useful in some patients, but he warned that in others it might make the pain much worse. He applied pressure to an area of the leg as a 'test' of the probable value of acupuncture in prospective patients. If this made the pain worse, he would not use it. In some people, he believed, the needles added to, rather than eased, the pain. In their case, perhaps, the acupuncture needles release into the circulation not an endorphin but a pain-heightening substance.

Dr Liem's observations are a strong support for the gate theory. We now know that the influences on the pain message as it travels from the site of the problem to the brain may worsen, rather than lessen, the brain's perception of pain. An essential part of the gate theory is that chemicals released within the brain itself may interfere with how it 'feels' pain, in either direction.

It might be thought here that I am dehumanizing pain, that I am trying to suggest that pain is a chemical and electrical phenomenon that is automatic, definable and measurable, and that is simply influenced by other chemical and electrical changes. That is quite wrong. The more we know about pain, the more we realize that our perception of pain, our reactions to it, and how much we are disabled by it, depend very much on our mood and emotional state at the time, our mental attitudes to it, and the way we behave when we have pain.

Melzack and Wall continued to develop and expand their gate theory over the years. By 1996, their concept was no longer of a sort of telephone line ascending from the periphery of the body to the brain, but of a computer-like network connecting the nerves, the spinal cord and the brain in many ways and in all directions. Each branch of the network has the potential to change how we feel pain (Melzack, 1996, pp. 128–38; Wall, 1996, pp. 15–22). A strong support for this explanation of pain is the finding from modern brain imaging techniques that, contrary to previous belief, there is no special 'pain centre' within the brain. Virtually the whole brain is involved in the perception of pain. This is good evidence that pain involves the whole person, and that the best approach to the management of pain should be many-faceted, involving mental as well as physical techniques.

So how does the modern doctor view pain? First of all, and most important, pain is what we feel in our brain, or our mind, if that is how we define consciousness. It is not just an automatic reaction to some painful event impinging on our bodies. In fact, we can feel pain when there is no obvious stimulus for it, and when there is no physical evidence for damage, disease or inflammation in the place where we feel the pain. It is a mental state, first and foremost. When we lose consciousness, as under an anaesthetic, we can no longer feel pain.

Second, pain is real. It is not imagined. If people say they are in pain, they are in pain. It isn't separable into mental or physical pain. If pain is such that it distresses you, then it is severe pain, regardless of whether that amount of pain might not distress another person so much. The average person would feel much more pain in a boxing ring against Mike Tyson than Lennox Lewis does, although the punch that delivered the pain is just the same.

Third, pain has an emotional aspect to it that differs from person to person. It is obviously an experience that you have in a particular part of the body, so that it is a physical activity, but it is always unpleasant, and therefore is an emotional experience too. We can, though, do something about our emotional response to pain. The extreme example is masochism, in which people can actually turn pain into a pleasure. I don't recommend this to anyone, but people have learned to control the emotional aspect of pain so that it is more bearable: some Eastern religions make this a part of their way of life.

Fourth, the way we react to pain can make a big difference to how we feel it. Do we tense up, grimace, weep, become immobile, and angry? Or do we act the stoic – put a brave face on it, try to shrug it off, and work on? How we react to pain has a considerable influence on whether we can carry on with normal life or not. It does not seem to be linked in a direct way to the severity of the pain or to the disease or injury that is causing it.

Fifth, once we have had a bout of pain, we may fear the next. That fear itself can make how we react to it worse. If we are worried about future pain, then when it does arrive we may tolerate it less well than if we can 'take it in our stride'. Being afraid of pain that hasn't yet come can be so great that it becomes an illness in itself, and one that badly damages our quality of life.

Sixth, when we are in pain, it is almost impossible for us to find accurate words to describe it to someone else. Our language just doesn't have the words, and in the emotional turmoil of acute pain, we are not at our best in finding them. So it is incumbent on everyone caring for people in pain to be patient and understanding. At times that isn't easy, especially if emotions are running high for both patient and carer.

Finally, there is acute pain and chronic pain. They are distinct, almost separate, entities that need different approaches. Acute pain is defined as a short-term attack of pain – perhaps the sort of pain you get when you have lifted something awkwardly, and that then persists over a few hours or days. Chronic pain is the persistent pain that continues, night and day, for weeks or months, long after the event that may have initiated it has been forgotten. Doctors have argued about the time of transition from 'acute' to 'chronic', but they seem to have decided upon six weeks or so. We expect a bout of acute sciatica to settle within that time.

The difference between the two is crucial. In acute pain the injury that has caused it is still present. Muscles may still be bruised and in a state of spasm or cramp. You are 'poleaxed' by it, so that you can't do anything else while you have it. The treatment of such pain is aimed not just at easing the pain, but at correcting, if possible, the injury or inflammation and relieving any cramp. Stretching the right muscles may be all that is needed. People with acute pain are often, understandably, very anxious, and that must be treated too. Constant reassurance that it will go, and that it is not a sign of serious illness, helps.

In contrast, in chronic pain the initial injury or illness has almost always healed. You struggle on with your daily routine while suffering this chronic pain, but it impinges on almost every aspect of your life. The aim here is to treat the pain and the disability that accompanies it. There is no damage or injury to correct, and anxiety has been replaced, almost invariably, and equally understandably, by depression. This does not mean that chronic pain is less real than acute pain, but it does mean that it is different, and carries with it different implications and a different approach to treatment. It is usually far easier to treat acute pain successfully than it is to cure chronic pain. As chronic pain persists, it disturbs sleep, and with that come the other symptoms of depression, such as lack of enjoyment in life, loss of appetite, and often an inward-looking withdrawal from contacts with friends and family.

Chronic pain is very destructive, emotionally as well as physically, and people with it need to be given hope and encouragement, as well as adequate treatment for their pain. They need to be helped to become more active mentally, as well as physically, so that they can return to their previously normal lifestyle. No one who treats people with chronic back pain can do so adequately unless they attend to their mental as well as their physical state.

Dividing pain into acute and chronic is useful, but it doesn't always fit with the experience of back-pain sufferers. Most people with back pain have repeated attacks of the pain, each of which could be described as acute. However, there comes a time when repeated attacks of pain merge into a chronic state, with a constant underlying discomfort that at times becomes acute. Defining a pain as repeatedly acute or as chronic is an academic exercise that may be of interest to researchers, but is of little import to people with pain.

Assessing your pain

What people with pain really need is evidence that their treatment will cure it. Today's doctors must practise evidence-based medicine. Before trying a new treatment or, for that matter, continuing with an old treatment, whether with drugs or physical methods, trials must have shown objective evidence that they are effective and safe. We must be able to put numbers on our assessment of pain, so that it can be amenable to analysis.

Dr Melzack, of gate theory fame (see page 15), has tackled this problem with his McGill Pain Questionnaire (Melzack, 1987, pp. 191–7). He divides the words used for pain into those that describe the physical feeling and those that describe its emotional effects.

In the first category are words such as throbbing, shooting, stabbing, sharp, cramp, gnawing, burning, aching, heaviness, tenderness and splitting. In the second are words like tiring, exhausting, sickening, fearful, punishing and cruel. The questionnaire lists all these categories in order, and asks you to 'tick', for each of them, boxes labelled none, mild, moderate and severe. At the bottom of the questionnaire, there is a 10-centimetre line, with, at the left end of it, the words 'no pain', and at the right end of it, the words 'worst possible pain'. You are asked to mark a spot along this line that you consider to be your severity of pain. To complete the questionnaire, there is a 'present pain intensity' assessment, on which you are asked to judge the pain you feel at the moment of completing the questionnaire. This is a scale from 0 to 5: 0 being no pain, 1 mild, 2 discomforting, 3 distressing, 4 horrible, and 5 excruciating. All the numbers from all three aspects of the questionnaire are added together to give a total score.

The results are a surprisingly accurate depiction of your pain. They are invaluable in giving doctors an objective idea of how bad your pain is before treatment. Because it allows every aspect of your pain to be represented as a number, it has become the standard tool for mathematical analysis of the difference that treatments can make to pain, and how they compare. You can use this questionnaire yourself, say, from month to month, to see if your chronic pain or repeated acute pain is improving or worsening, and in which ways, and by how much. You may find from completing it that relying on your memory of your pain is not as accurate as you thought. However, it does not make any reference to how badly the pain has interfered with your ability to live normally. That is at least as important, though, as the pain itself, and needs another type of assessment.

Assessing the disability caused by someone's pain

Treating the pain, although vital, is not enough. As most people with back pain are restricted in some physical and/or mental way by it, we also need to restore them to as near to normal life as possible. Just as we need to assess someone's pain objectively, we need to do the same with their disability. Only then can we gauge whether the treatment is helping enough.

Here I must refer again to my favourite back-pain man, Professor Waddell who, with his colleague and clinical psychologist Dr Chris Main of Salford, established the standards for assessing the disability that is linked with back pain. They asked their subjects to give yes or no answers to the following questions:

- Do you need help for, or avoid, lifting a weight of 30 pounds or so, such as a heavy suitcase or a three-year-old child?
- Can you sit in an ordinary chair for 30 minutes without having to get up and move around?
- Can you stand in one place for 30 minutes before having to move?
- Can you walk for 30 minutes, or for up to 2 miles, without needing to rest?
- Can you travel in a car or bus for 30 minutes without the need for a break?
- Do you often miss, or have to leave early, social activities that other people find no problem?
- Is your sleep disturbed by pain twice or three times a week or more?
- Have you reduced or stopped your sex life because it gives you pain?
- Do you need help to put on or take off shoes, socks or tights, or to tie and untie shoelaces?

A more complex questionnaire widely used by doctors in assessing disability due to back pain was published by Roland and Morris in 1983 (Roland and Morris, 1983, pp. 141–4). It asks people with back pain to tick the following 24 statements if they apply to them.
Because of my back pain:

1 I stay at home most of the time.
2 I change position frequently.
3 I walk more slowly than usual.
4 I am not doing the jobs I usually do around the house.
5 I use a handrail to go upstairs.
6 I lie down to rest more often than before.
7 I have to hold on to something to get out of an easy chair.
8 I try to get other people to do things for me.
9 I get dressed more slowly than usual.
10 I only stand for short periods.

11 I try not to bend or kneel.
12 I find it difficult to get out of a chair.
13 I am in pain most of the time.
14 I find it difficult to turn over in bed.
15 I have lost my appetite.
16 I have trouble putting on socks or stockings.
17 I only walk short distances.
18 I sleep less well than before.
19 I need help to dress myself.
20 I sit down for most of the day.
21 I avoid heavy jobs around the house.
22 I am more irritable and bad tempered than I used to be.
23 I go upstairs more slowly than before.
24 I stay in bed most of the time.

Although the answers to these two questionnaires are subjective, in that they rely on people's own reports of their problems, taken together they form a practical and reliable baseline on which to judge treatments and progress. They are the standard tests by which judgements on new treatments are made.

Of course, answers to questionnaires cannot stand alone as the sole measure of your disability. Your doctor will need a more objective assessment of how your back is functioning. A standard test for this is the 'shuttle walk'. You will be asked to walk along a 10-metre path, which has a cone a half-metre from each end. Your task is to walk round the cones, back and forward along the path at a starting speed of 30 metres (in effect, one and a half 'laps') in one minute. Every minute you are asked to speed up by 10 metres a minute, so that you reach a rate of 140 metres per minute by the twelfth minute. The test is stopped when you become too tired, or your back pain becomes too much, or the examiner decides you have not met the required speed. The result is recorded as the total number of metres you have managed to walk.

Fogg and Taylor (Fogg and Taylor, 1997) presented this test to the International Society for the Study of the Lumbar Spine in its Annual Conference in Singapore in 1997, and showed it to be a sensitive and efficient way to measure the response of back pain to treatment. Patients responding to treatment found they could quickly improve their walking distances and times.

Of course, there is one caveat to all this. Questionnaires and shuttle walks are fine if the patient is honest and wants to do well and get better. They can even help people to motivate themselves to improve their performance. Discovering that your questionnaire scores are falling and your walk speeds and times are improving can be a big boost to confidence and to feeling better. Unfortunately, though, there still remain some people who make back pain an excuse to avoid major problems in their family life and at work. They may even see their pain as a way of making money through litigation about its supposed or actual cause. People who are on this tack will do badly in both questionnaires and shuttle walks, and there is little that their doctors can do for them. Some do seem to become suddenly better when their compensation claims are settled. It is very difficult for doctors to recognize such people, and differentiate them from the vast majority, for whom absolutely the worst thing about back pain is that they need to take time off work and lose much-needed income – and may even lose their jobs in some cases.

We therefore assume, charitably, that everyone is in the latter category. It is for all those people that the next chapters are meant.

4

Back pain – who gets it and why

Back pain is almost normal, in that most of us get it at some time in our lives. It affects men and women equally. The patterns of pain between the sexes may differ a little, so that men are slightly more likely than women to have sciatica, and more women complain of a general backache than men. Back pain peaks between the ages of 40 and 60 – the later working years – so that for many middle-aged adults it seems to wear off, or at least be less of a problem, as they age. Unfortunately, in those who continue to have back pain beyond middle age, the attacks become more frequent, and chronic pain becomes more persistent as they grow older.

There are plenty of myths about back pain that need to be dispelled. For example, back pain does not afflict people of a particular height, weight or body shape. So being overweight – or even frankly obese – does not make men or women more prone than others to suffer back pain. Much as I would like to devote a chapter to the need to lose weight, there is no need. Losing excess weight does not appear to make a difference to back pain – although it does, of course, lower the risks of other diseases such as heart attacks, and make you fitter too. There is some evidence that being fitter can help you recover faster and more completely from low back pain, but it does not appear to prevent you having an initial attack.

On the other hand, many highly sophisticated studies have reported that smokers have more back pain than non-smokers, and that the pain is worse the more tobacco they consume. Many explanations are offered for this. One is that people who smoke differ from non-smokers in other health-related habits and in their psychology and social behaviour, all of which may affect back pain. There are also good reasons for linking smoking directly with back pain. It causes a chronic cough, which can put pressure on discs, possibly making them bulge and press on nerves in the back. Nicotine is also a powerful constrictor of blood vessels, so that it reduces the blood flow to the back tissues. Discs need all the oxygen that they can get to diffuse into them (they have no blood vessels inside them) so that any reduction of flow to the back tissues puts them at risk. This has been graphically illustrated in animal studies, which have shown that smoking directly damages the intervertebral discs.

The best evidence that smoking damages human discs was given by Battie and his colleagues in 1991 (Battie and colleagues, 1991, pp. 1015–21). They studied a series of identical twins, each set comprising one smoking and one non-smoking twin. MRI scans of the discs of the smokers showed significantly more degeneration than those of their non-smoking twins. Their study supported the results of a 1989 study by Deyo and Bass (Deyo and Bass, 1989, pp. 501–6). Working on the records of very large numbers of people in the United States, they found that people smoking more than 60 cigarettes a day had much more back pain than the rest of the population The pain must ease when people stop smoking, because those who had smoked, but stopped more than ten years before the study, had no more back pain than people who had never smoked.

It has to be concluded that if you have back pain and smoke, you should stop. It will not only prove a good move for your general health, it will probably reduce your pain.

The type of work we do also influences whether or not we are likely to have back pain. But it isn't a simple relationship. It isn't simply a matter of heavy physical work equating to back injury and therefore pain. It is true that many cases of acute – and later chronic – back pain can be traced to one incident when (or after which) the person felt 'something go' in the back, and the pain either started then or some hours later.

The causes of such pain have been listed as:

- regular heavy manual work;
- lifting;
- twisting;
- sitting for long periods;
- driving.

So do these activities really cause a lot of back pain? It is very difficult to prove it. The most recent surveys show that manual and sedentary workers have a similar frequency of attacks of back pain enough to make them take time off work. The manual workers stay off a little longer with each episode. However, this may be more to do with the nature of their jobs – sedentary workers may be able to return sooner because their jobs allow them to return when there is still a residual pain. That could be impossible for a person who needs to be physically fitter to do his job. My own experience tells me that I would keep a manual worker off work longer than, say, an office worker, after similar episodes of back injury or pain.

Lifting heavy weights certainly causes many episodes of back pain. However, even this is not as clear-cut as it appears. Despite many efforts to link lifting with back pain, few researchers have come to definite conclusions. There is almost universal agreement among them that repeated lifting of less than around 11 kilograms (25 pounds) does not cause backache. But is there any real evidence that repeatedly lifting more than that causes back pain? MacFarlane and his colleagues set up the South Manchester Study to look into what sort of physical work might lead to back pain. They published their conclusions in 1997 (MacFarlane and colleagues, 1997, pp. 1143–9). Their findings seemed to show that whatever type of job the men in their study did had no effect on whether they would develop back pain. However, there was a difference among the women in the study. Women doing shift work whose jobs entailed standing and walking about for more than two hours, or who lifted and moved weights over 11 kilograms (25 pounds), were marginally more likely to have back pain than those who remained seated and did little heavy work. There was no increase in back pain in men or women who had been in such jobs longer, or as they grew older. So we cannot use the South Manchester Study for evidence to blame heavy work for most back pain.

Theoretically, combining lifting with bending and twisting, or over-reaching with the back muscles, should be a common cause of pain. Yet there are no reliable studies confirming this. Many people link their back pain with long periods of sitting awkwardly in a poor unsupported position. Once again, though, there is no evidence that sitting for long periods, regardless of the position, can actually initiate back pain, but it may worsen a back pain that is already present for other reasons.

There is probably a link between long periods of driving and back pain. At least two well-organized studies have concluded that people who spend a lot of time driving are more likely to have back trouble than people who don't (Troup, 1978, pp. 207–14; Hulshof and van Zanten, 1987, pp. 205–20).

Why should driving be more likely to cause the pain than, say, heavy work? The clue may lie in the fact that cars and other vehicles

27

vibrate at around the same frequency as the natural resonance of the spine. (For the technically minded, this is 4-6 Hz.) Constant exposure to this vibration, which we probably hardly notice, is enough, in theory, to cause the spine and discs to vibrate in sympathy – and this is enough to speed up the degeneration of the structure of the bones that we have to expect as we age (Pope and colleagues, 1991, pp. 1487–1501). The lesson from this is to try to eliminate vibration from your vehicle – and this is not so easy as it sounds. If you have constant back pain and drive for a living, you should consider changing your occupation.

Then there is the minefield of repetitive strain injury, commonly known as RSI. Traditionally, RSI claims have concentrated on the wrist, and have been made by keyboard operators. The debate still rages between the people who are sure that it exists and those who see it as a way of getting compensation for their unhappiness at work. I definitely do not wish to take sides on that one. However, claims that RSI might affect back muscles are also rising. Could back pain be caused by repeated movements of the back at work?

As with RSI of the wrist, the concept of a back pain RSI is a matter of hot debate. The problem for its supporters is that to reproduce failure of the back muscles (which is presumably the mechanism of RSI) in the research laboratory, you need to expose them to far faster and many more activities of use than could even be asked for, or achieved, at work. There is no real evidence that repeated use of back muscles at work causes RSI in the back. As with lifting and twisting, repeated movements of the back may worsen a backache that is already there, but they do not seem to be its fundamental cause.

So if none of these activities cause back pain, you will be wondering by now what on earth does? Could it be largely psychological? Is it all in the mind? I'm sure that particular suggestion will raise your hackles. It is very unfair, and indeed insulting, to suggest to anyone with back pain that they are imagining their pain, and I certainly do not want to suggest that in any way. I repeat what was written in the last chapter: all pain is real, and if you say you have it, you have it.

So why am I bringing in the subject of the mind? Let's go back to evidence-based medicine. In the 1970s, reports of studies of working populations, to begin with in Scandinavia, suggested that people in monotonous jobs and with little satisfaction in their work, who felt their bosses didn't care, went 'off sick' with back pain more often and for longer than others. Then came the Boeing study that followed, over a four-year period, 3,000 aircraft workers, who were apparently normal, with no back pain, before the study started. The idea was to find 'predictors' in their physical and mental make-up that would indicate who would develop back pain during the study.

It turned out that differences in physique, fitness and strength had no influence on whether or not people developed back pain. Psychological problems and job dissatisfaction were very weak predictors of back pain, but could only account for around 3 per cent of cases. This result has been supported since by a study in 8,000 Finnish farmers, in which those with some mental stress seemed to be a little more likely than others to develop back pain, and, once again, that physique or previous injuries made no difference (Manninen and colleagues, 1995, p. 37). A series of other studies, too many to mention here, have come to similar conclusions. The main finding in one was that mental stress and job dissatisfaction can induce chronic back pain, but only in a small minority of all the cases of back pain. When these things are the cause, the pain is always vague, and unrelated to disc problems and nerve root pain. Stress and unhappiness at work do cause back pain, but not physical disease in the spine.

What can we conclude about the causes of back pain from all these reports? First is the fact that most of us, male or female, get back pain at some time in our lives. It doesn't matter how tall or short we are, or how fat or thin. Nor does it seem to matter how much physical work we do. Although many people believe that heavy physical work causes what they think of as 'wear and tear' in the back, there is little or no evidence that it does. In fact, the evidence is growing that physical work strengthens and protects the back against pain. At times, tackling a heavier job than usual for you can cause back pain, but it is usually fleeting and does not lead to chronic back pain or to repeated episodes of acute back pain. On the whole, hard work is good, not bad, for your back.

So when people are told they have back pain because 'their back is too long' or 'their legs are of unequal length', or they are too tall, too short, too fat, or too thin, there is no evidence to support these statements. More than that, such advice can do harm, because if people believe that these are the causes of their pain, they can become convinced that nothing can be done about it. They can do little about their size and build, so they accept that their pain is inevitable and untreatable. This is the first step to becoming an unemployable permanent invalid. And that is a disastrous mistake.

Telling people with back pain to stay off work and rest until it eases off can be just as harmful. Rest can make things worse – when in fact the opposite, muscle activity, is needed. Even worse is to advise them to change their job for a lighter one. It is hardly ever possible to blame a backache on a job, or to state categorically that a job is bad for an already bad back, or that a lighter job would cure the pain. When people change jobs for these reasons, the new job is almost always more poorly paid, and if the pain persists, it is soon seen as a mistake. This often leads to resentment and even further dissatisfaction in life – which makes the pain even worse. You enter a vicious cycle from which it is difficult to escape. So before you take the decision to change your life in a major way because you have back pain, think hard. You may not have acquired that back pain through your job, and you may regret, in the future, needlessly giving up a career, a sport or a hobby.

Keep an open mind about your back pain until you have read the next few chapters. They may well make a difference to your decisions about your future, and not just about your back pain.

5
Patterns of back pain

Ask 500 people with back pain how it started. How do you think they will respond? Professor Waddell did precisely that in his clinic in Scotland. Around 300 (60 per cent) said it started suddenly: for the others, it was a gradual process. Most of the 'sudden' group felt that the event that precipitated the pain for the first time was a normal action like lifting or bending, one that they had performed many times before. However, few could pinpoint the cause of their most recent attack of acute pain, and even fewer could say that any particular activity was the cause of repeated attacks of pain. They just arrived, virtually 'out of the blue'.

Contrast these replies with the details given by almost 8,000 people attending the Canadian Back Institute (Hall and colleagues, 1998, p. 2). Of those who looked after their own health care, and were not in litigation about their pain, two-thirds could not say what had initiated it. Of those who were aiming for compensation for their pain or were suing employers, 91 per cent blamed a particular incident for it. I leave the reader to draw their own conclusions about this finding. Suffice it to say that it is often difficult to know where to put the blame for each episode of pain.

Given that it is difficult to be sure what has caused the bout of back pain, is the average bout of back pain predictable, in its course and timing? The medical schools think so. They teach students that between three-quarters and 90 per cent of people who develop an episode of acute back pain are better within six weeks. Most return to work within that time. However, these are results from specialist clinics. GPs see back pain from a different perspective.

The South Manchester Study followed people treated by their family doctors for back pain. Most (69 per cent) were seen in a new attack, one in five were in an acute phase of a chronic pain, and 8 per cent had chronic pain. Of them all, only 27 per cent were completely better within three months: 28 per cent had improved, and 30 per cent were still complaining of the same pain. Some 14 per cent were actually worse.

Many other studies have reported similar results. By around four weeks, most people who see their family doctors for back pain are much better, but they are not usually free of pain. Around a quarter of them are still substantially disabled by their pain. However, after one year, around 70 per cent still have back problems, a third of whom have fairly severe persistent pain. Around one in five are still disabled to some degree by their pain, in that they are restricted in their movements and activities.

So, assuming that you are in your first episode of acute back pain, what would be a fair prediction about how you will progress? You can be reassured that, no matter how you are treated (or even not treated), your pain is almost certainly going to lessen over the next few weeks. You can probably stay at work or can go back to work within a week or so, even if you continue to have some pain. You can expect other acute episodes of back pain in the future, which may eventually disappear in time.

You may also have to accept that some cases of acute back pain can become chronic, but that your medical team will do its best to prevent that. Even if your pain does become chronic, it is likely to disappear eventually. Be reassured that most people with back pain can continue with a normal life, in spite of their pain.

Of course, faced with that first episode of pain, you will want to know whether you are among the fortunate majority whose pain will go fairly soon, or are among the few whose pain will persist and recur, so that you become classified as having repeated acute pain or persistent chronic pain. This is where you may become angry with me again, but don't shoot the messenger because his message is not palatable.

The facts are fairly clear, following the analysis of many studies. Remember the classification of back pain in Chapter 1 into the three groups of simple pain, nerve root pain and serious spinal disease? Remember, too, that the last two categories only account for around 5 per cent of all back pain. If you are unlucky enough to be in one of them, then your pain is likely to persist beyond a few weeks. You will probably need treatment for your underlying problem before it clears up.

If you are in the 95 per cent whose back pain is classified as simple, then it may persist beyond a month or so if your initial pain was more severe than usual. This will take longer to settle, but should still clear up within six weeks. People who take longer than that are likely to believe that their back pain is caused by their work, or are under considerable mental stress, or are unhappy at work.

They may be actively seeking compensation or want more time off work because they can't face going back. The longer a person is off work with back pain, the less likely he or she is to go back at all.

This is where you may start to get angry, but the facts from a lot of good studies show that doctors can't predict from their initial examination of the back, or from the pain's initial severity, whether or not you will have long-term pain. But they can predict just that from your attitude to the pain, and if you think it is work-related. In particular, if you blame your employer, directly or indirectly, for your pain, it has a much higher chance of persisting and becoming a chronic back pain that is very difficult to manage and cure.

This doesn't mean that most people with long-term back pain are malingerers. They have real pain that is influenced by their emotional and mental stresses. But it does mean that to manage their long-term back pain successfully, they may have to change their mental attitudes to their pain – and, in some cases, lose their determination to make as much money from it as they can. In assigning blame to the cause of the pain, and particularly in pursuing some redress for it, they are in danger of perpetuating their problems, and of becoming invalids who are unable to fit well again into society – whether this be work, or good relationships with their friends and family. If you are involved in a lawsuit about the cause of your back pain, it may be far better and healthier for you to drop it, find other work, and get on with your life. You won't be constantly in a state of anger, you will be able to relax more, and it may also cure the pain.

6
The mechanisms of back pain

Let's concentrate in this chapter on the vast majority of cases of back pain: those with simple back pain that is not caused by nerve root pressure or by serious spinal disease. Which structure in the back is actually aching?

It is a common assumption that if we are in pain there must be something wrong with some structure or tissue. For example, it is assumed that a bone may be out of place, or a joint swollen, or a muscle fibre or ligament torn, or pressure is put on a nerve by a swollen disc. It is true that all these can cause pain, but how often do they do so? And in what proportion of people with back pain can any of these problems be identified as the cause of the pain? The answer is very few. Most people with back pain have backs that are structurally normal. Their spines are straight, and all the joints between the vertebrae are in their proper position and are not swollen or inflamed. There is no evidence of torn muscles or ligaments, or of bulging discs pressing upon nerves. Yet their back pain is very real.

This is not to say their muscles are necessarily 'normal', that is, the same as everyone else's muscles. Muscles strengthen with repeated use and weaken when they are under-used. So people with different lifestyles and occupations may use their back muscles differently. The relative strengths and bulk of their muscles eventually differ, so the back muscles in people who do a lot of physical work are quite different from those who sit most of the time. Stronger muscles cope with exercise better than weaker muscles, which on unusual exertion can become easily tired, or become swollen, tender and go easily into cramp, or spasm. That leads to a very painful back.

So do not be surprised, even if your back pain is fairly severe, when you are told that there is nothing fundamentally wrong with your back. Your pain may be due to repeated muscle fatigue, because your muscles are unable to cope with the load you are putting upon them.

This may be a difficult concept to deal with, as the accepted wisdom for many years has been that back pain must mean 'something wrong in the back'. Whole systems of back-pain management depend on twisting, tweaking, jerking, stretching and even operating on backs because the joints in the spine are 'out of alignment'. Often such manipulations are very successful, but I would submit that all that is happening is that muscles in cramp are being stretched, and therefore relaxed. Stretch a cramped muscle and the pain goes, instantly. As we said before, if you have cramp in the calf, all you need to do to relieve it is to pull up your foot. Cramp in the sole of the foot is relieved by pulling on the relevant toe. Cramp in the back is relieved by stretching the appropriate muscle – and a good stretch is a good way to do it.

If you find it difficult to accept that your pain in the back is not linked to any physical abnormality of your spine or the structures around it, I would refer you again to Professor Waddell's brilliant book, *The Back Pain Revolution*. He shows his patients very simply how fatigue in a normal muscle can cause a lot of pain.

He asks them to make four 'observations':

1 The first is to hold a weight of a few pounds at arm's length, the hand being at around shoulder height. After only a few minutes it hurts, the pain spreading along the arm from shoulder to hand. Shortly afterwards, you have to put the weight down.

2 The second is to rest one elbow on a table with your forearm vertical. With a straight hand and fingers, bend back your wrist, then use your other hand to bend back your middle finger as far as it will go. Keep it there. Your finger soon becomes painful, and you have to let it go.

3 The third observation is that the pain of cramp continues until you manage to stretch and relax the affected muscle.

4 The fourth is that if we try to exercise hard after we have let ourselves become unfit, our muscles and joints ache and swell much more than they did when we were fitter. The pain in the muscles can persist for days afterwards.

Professor Waddell makes the point that these observations apply to everyone: they do not depend on having muscle or joint damage or misalignment. He calls the mechanism behind this sort of pain 'dysfunction', and he is convinced that dysfunction lies behind most cases of back pain. I agree with him wholeheartedly.

Apply these four observations to most people with back pain.

Take observations 1 and 2. At some time you may have put your back muscles into a position, or asked them to do a task, that involved the equivalent of holding a weight for a long period. Perhaps you were standing awkwardly, with your spine twisted, while holding a heavy weight. Or were carrying a load with one hand, so that your spine was bent towards that side. After only a few minutes, it would become painful, so that you had to put the load down and transfer it to the other hand. That would ease the pain, for it to reappear after a few minutes on the load-bearing side. There is no need to postulate an injury to the muscles to explain the pain. You are doing to the back what you did to your arms and fingers in the first two observations – you asked your muscles to bear too much weight for too long, and by bending your spine you asked them to stretch for too long.

Now take observation 3. Think about what happens after carrying the weight: the backache persists for hours afterwards. Resting the back doesn't help: in fact, it makes the pain worse as the back muscles stiffen. But walking about and stretching the back helps a lot. In effect, you are stretching the cramp out of the muscles. Then, and only then, can you relax them. Once again, think of the last time you had cramp, say, in your calf muscle. You could only relieve it by pulling up your foot, stretching the muscle. The same goes for the back.

Then there is observation 4. Most of us are fairly unfit. I apologize in advance to you if you are an athlete in training, but I suspect that if you were, you wouldn't be reading this book. But let's assume that it is a long time since you did regular physical exercise, or even broke into a run. Then you decide to do something physical, like digging the garden. For several days afterwards your muscles, probably all of them, will ache and feel swollen. They are just trying to adapt to the new load you have put upon them. And while they do, they are swollen and painful. This is a normal change in your muscles. They are not 'torn' or 'sprained' or 'strained' – and nor are your ligaments or joints. If you increase your exercise so that you are doing the equivalent of digging the garden every day, your muscles will get used to the extra exercise, and won't complain. They will adapt. But if you only exercise intermittently, you can expect repeated aches and pains in your muscles. This is 'dysfunction'.

Accepting dysfunction as the cause of back pain brings both good and bad news for sufferers. The good news is that, because there is no underlying disease of the back, it can be treated very successfully, with the hope that most people with back pain will recover completely. The bad news is that the symptoms will persist if the circumstances leading to the dysfunction are not dealt with. Most of the rest of this book, which concentrates on how you can help to ease your own back pain, is based on the need to correct the dysfunction in the muscles of your back, which are essentially normal.

Before you read on, however, you need to know how muscles work. We human beings, although now civilized, are still physically essentially hunter-gatherers. To keep fit we need to use our muscles. We must continue to be physically active throughout our lives, not just to keep our muscles efficient and our bones strong, but to keep our nervous systems at peak performance and to improve our tolerance of pain. If we stop exercising – in effect, become couch potatoes – our muscles deteriorate, and our hearts and nervous systems suffer. We become more sensitive to pain. The medical word for this is 'deconditioning'.

According to sports medicine specialists Mayer and Gatchel, deconditioning plays a large part in causing back pain and the disability that it produces (Mayer and Gatchel, 1988). They found that people with long-term chronic back pain have lost much of their ability to move their spines, have much weaker back muscles, their hearts are much less able to tolerate exercise, and they are much less able than others to lift objects. Mayer and Gatchel claim that these problems are all caused by lack of use of the back muscles: they treat back pain with vigorous exercise, aiming to restore the normal muscle systems in the back.

Their approach certainly seems to work. In the past it was common for doctors to recommend bed rest for many illnesses. The idea was that rest allowed the body to heal without expending unnecessary energy in exercise. For example, in the 1960s, medical students were taught that the best way to help people recover from a heart attack was to make them lie flat in a bed for at least six weeks, and preferably longer, before allowing them even to sit up, far less exercise again. It was thought then that the heart muscle would heal with a stronger scar if it was not exposed to the extra demands that exercise would put upon it.

This turned out to be exactly the opposite of what was really needed. Today we allow people to get out of bed within the first few days after a heart attack, and encourage exercise to make the heart muscle fitter and to encourage it to heal more firmly. Bed rest is hardly ever recommended for even the most serious illnesses. Here is a list of the unwanted effects of rest in bed for long periods. It leads to:

- loss of muscle;
- loss of minerals from bone, making it weaker;
- stiffness due to loss of range of movement in joints and to thickening of the tissues around the joints;
- shortening of the time before reaching muscle fatigue and exhaustion when exercising;
- loss of the co-ordination between muscles and the nervous system;
- loss of ligament strength;
- slower healing;
- poorer general fitness, especially of the heart;
- greater susceptibility to anaemia and clotting;
- a less effective immune system with lowered resistance to infection;
- dulling of the senses and of the intellect;
- mental distress and depression;
- a lower tolerance to pain.

So bed rest for back pain is not an option, no matter how comforting it may be in the short term. The real best choice for the patient is to 'recondition' the back. Our problem as doctors is how to get this idea across in the most understandable way to our patients, who are convinced that they have a problem with a disc or a 'trapped nerve'. If you think you have an abnormal disc or nerve problem, you naturally believe it is unlikely to correct itself, and that you need to rest or undergo surgery for it.

This is very rarely the case. If you could take just two messages from this book, the first is that most people with back pain have no underlying disease or damage or joint misalignment or displacement in their spines. Their backs are just not working efficiently, and are therefore 'complaining' to them by causing pain. If this applies to you, then you will recognize the following picture of yourself. You may be standing or sitting incorrectly: you may be stiff and less flexible than before, finding it less easy to move around freely. Your muscles may be weak and you may tire quickly. You may find it difficult to control your movements as well, so that your balance and co-ordination are disturbed. You may be more sensitive to pain than you were. You may become anxious as all these symptoms pile up on you.

The second message is that the treatment of your pain should be aimed at correcting all of these problems. It doesn't really matter what caused your back pain in the first place: you must deal with your back as it is now. The best way to do that is to get your back moving normally again. The only person who can do that is you. Your doctor, physiotherapist, chiropractor or osteopath cannot do it for you.

7
Reconditioning your back (1) – what can be done by your doctor for acute back pain

The biggest debate among doctors, GPs and specialists about the treatment of back pain used to be whether the patient should rest or be active. However, this was settled beyond dispute by three large trials in the 1980s and 1990s which showed that people with sciatica and other forms of low back pain who stayed active, rather than rested, had fewer recurrences of pain and had less time off work in the following year. Two of them showed very conclusively that they also recovered from the pain faster than those who had been told to rest (Lindequist and colleagues, 1984, pp. 113–16; Linton and others, 1993, pp. 353–9; Lindstrom and colleagues, 1992, pp. 641–52).

The British Royal College of General Practitioners (RCGP) followed the publication of these trials with their own guidelines for family doctors. These are very straightforward, and very positive on the issue of 'exercising away' the pain. They are still in operation, and are summarized here:

The RCGP guidelines on the treatment of low back pain

Their conclusions after a review of all the trials:

- For acute or recurrent low back pain, with or without leg pain, bed rest for two to seven days is worse than placebo or normal activity. It is not as effective as other treatments in relieving pain, speed of recovery, return to normal daily activities or days lost from work.
- Longer bed rest may lead to weakness, chronic debility and increased difficulty in being rehabilitated into work.
- Advice to continue ordinary activity leads to better recovery from an acute attack of back pain and to less time off work than the traditional advice of rest.

40

- A gradual return to normal activities over a few days, along with advice on how to manage pain, leads to less eventual disability than the advice to rest.
- It also leads to less time off work.

Their recommendations – doctors should:

- Not recommend or use rest as a treatment for back pain.
- Advise patients to stay as active as possible and to continue normal activities even when they have pain.
- Advise patients to increase their activities progressively.
- Advise patients to stay at work or get back to work as soon as possible, as this is medically beneficial to them.

The guidelines add that although some patients go to bed because of their pain, this should not be looked upon as a form of treatment.

So the goals of treatment are clear. If you have back pain you must work through it, rather than lie down with it. That is all very well, but sometimes the pain seems too much to be able to do anything but surrender to it. It is all very well saying to people to get up and be active, but how do they do it? This is what the rest of the book is about.

The first problem with the RCGP's advice is that the extra activity may eventually get the back working again, but it doesn't immediately address the main problem – the pain itself. More activity may initially make the pain worse, so the first priority is to ease the pain, and the second is to recondition the back, so that the pain doesn't recur.

Drugs for pain

The first step on the road to recovery is to take drugs to kill the pain – analgesics. The two main ones in use today are aspirin and paracetamol. There are dozens of different combinations of drugs to ease pain that can be bought from pharmacies or prescribed by doctors, but the basis of most of them remains an adequate dose of either of these two drugs. For aspirin, this is two or three tablets of 300 mg every four hours, and for paracetamol, it is two tablets of 500 mg every four hours, but no more than four times a day. The timing is vital. You should not wait until the pain gets worse again before taking your next dose. For the first day or two after your back becomes painful, you should take the drugs every four hours, even if the last dose of the drug is still working when it is time to take the next. Painkiller drugs work much more effectively in preventing pain than in lessening pain once it is established.

'Non-Steroidal Anti-Inflammatory Drugs' (NSAIDs) are a development from aspirin. They include ibuprofen, naproxen, indomethacin, and diclofenac: there are many others. Like aspirin and paracetamol, they need to be given regularly to be most effective. There are no good trials proving they are more effective than aspirin or paracetamol, or that any NSAID is more effective than any other NSAID in back pain. Some seem to cause less stomach upsets than others.

There are plenty of painkiller tablets that combine aspirin or paracetamol with low doses of weak morphine-like drugs. Among them are co-codamol, co-dydramol and co-proxamol. They are names that are probably familiar to you, because they are among the most frequently prescribed painkillers by family doctors. Although useful in the early stages and probably somewhat more effective than either aspirin or paracetamol alone, they have the drawbacks that they can make you constipated and drowsy. People can also become dependent upon them, so that they eventually cannot do without them: this is not helpful, especially as this can affect someone's alertness at work and their leisure time with their families.

Muscle relaxants such as diazepam (Valium), baclofen and dantrolene have also been shown to ease back pain. They are not analgesics in themselves, but work by relieving cramp, which in turn eases pain. Unfortunately they too can cause sleepiness and dependence, even after only a few days. They are not recommended for more than the first few days, but all too many people with back pain eventually take them all the time. This is not good medicine.

Some people need injections to ease the pain in the first few days. Local anaesthetics, similar to those given in dental treatment, injected into the point where the pain is worst, can help for a while, but they are not recommended as a repeat cure for pain.

Two other forms of drug have been used for back pain, but there is no evidence that they are effective, and they are not recommended by the RCGP. One group includes the 'strong opioids' like morphine and codeine. They are no more effective in simple back pain than paracetamol or NSAIDs, yet they slow mental and nerve reactions, cause drowsiness, impair intellect, and can lead to dependence and addiction. The other group comprises the antidepressants. Among them are the 'tricyclics', such as amitriptyline (Lentizol, Triptafen) and imipramine (Tofranil) and the 'selective serotonin reuptake inhibitors', or SSRIs, which include paroxetine (Seroxat) and fluoxetine (Prozac). They may help lift a depression that is coincidental to, or that is linked to, the pain, but they do not directly ease the pain itself. As they too have a multitude of side effects, their possible benefits must be weighed against their drawbacks. For most people with uncomplicated back pain, the drawbacks heavily outweigh the benefits.

Now we come to the point that most people with back pain refuse to believe. It is that increasing activity doesn't worsen the pain. Instead, it decreases it. The problem is to work out the right type and amount of exercise for each person, and to accept that while it is a general rule that exercise helps, there may be a 'blip' or two, when the pain may get worse for a while, during the recovery period. Many people with pain are understandably frightened by the thought that increasing exercise will increase their pain, and their apprehension causes them to become more tense: that naturally causes more pain, and the fear becomes self-fulfilling.

By exercise is not meant specific exercises for the back muscles, but normal activity for the whole body. It means walking about, both on the flat and up and down inclines, or even stairs – all the activity that you normally undertake when your back is pain free. Treating back pain isn't just about the pain, it is about getting you back to normal. It is no use easing the pain, but leaving you in a permanent fear of the pain returning, or so dependent on rest as a treatment that you can never go back to work.

Treating the acute pain

Now it is time to become specific. So far I have written about principles, but we now have to face the reality of what to do for someone with an acute back pain. I am presuming here that the doctor has made sure that you have a 'simple' back pain, one that is not caused by pressure on a nerve or by serious disease of the spine and adjacent tissues. Remember that more than 95 per cent of cases of all acute back pain fall into this category. We will come to treatment of more serious causes of back pain later.

The first step is to be reassured. Although you may be in severe pain, you should accept that more than 90 per cent of acute back pains settle within, at most, six weeks, and often a lot sooner than that. You may also have to accept that you have more than an even chance (about 60 per cent) of having another episode of back pain in the next year. These recurrent attacks in the end will fade, so that most people will be free of them within three to five years of the first attack. And, as we have already stated, backache, thankfully, is not a problem that increases as we grow older: it has its peak incidence in the middle years, and is relatively rare from the fifties onward.

Of course, reassurance may help you worry less, and to relax, and in so doing may help relieve the spasm in cramped muscles. But it does not in itself ease pain. For this, the acute back-pain sufferer needs the effective painkillers that have already been listed. You may wish to discuss with your doctor which ones are suitable for you, and you may have to 'chop and change' a few times before you get the one that gives you the most relief. People differ a lot in their sensitivity to analgesics, and the medication that suits one person may not suit another. So if your pain is not being adequately relieved by one type of drug, ask for another. There should be one that works for you. Our general rule as family doctors is that if the patient needs painkillers regularly for more than two weeks, and the pain keeps resurfacing before the time for the next dose, we seek an urgent specialist opinion.

Manipulation

Next to be considered is manipulation, of which there are many types. It is practised by physiotherapists, osteopaths, chiropractors and some doctors such as myself. All are legitimate forms of treatment that have their supporters, despite the fact that they differ in the details of their manipulations. Muscles, spines and necks are stretched, bent, twisted and jerked, and the proponents of their own type of treatment, including doctors like myself, all have their own theories on how they work.

All I can say is that manipulation does work, and sometimes

dramatically. Patients come into the surgery bent over or to the side, in obvious pain and unable to walk or sit down, and leave the surgery walking straight and easily, and virtually free of their pain. It is very satisfying for both manipulator and 'manipulatee'. And I am not talking just about my own experience as a doctor who stretches backs. (I don't jerk or twist.) There are plenty of reports on how effective manipulation is for acute back pain.

As an aside, I can describe briefly what I do. Patients with acute sore backs arrive, usually limping, with the trunk angled to one side, and very stiff back muscles on that side. I first examine them standing up with their feet together, and ask them to bend forwards and backwards, then to each side, as far as they can. Standing behind them, I place my right foot beside their right foot and twist their shoulders around as far as I can. I do the same with my left foot.

This examination gives me a good idea of how stiff the back and torso muscles really are, and by how much the stiffness has restricted the person's movements. I then ask the patient to lie face down on the examination couch and put their hands behind the small of the back, with one hand gripping the wrist of the other. They then must arch their backs upwards, while pressing their hands into the back, at the same time trying to raise their knees off the couch. If they can hardly do this, I help them by pulling their shoulders straight upwards. It needs a lot of strength to do it, and can be uncomfortable for the patient.

I did not invent this exercise myself – it is one of Dr Cyriax's methods for relieving back spasm. Most of the time it works like a dream. The patient who has entered the room bent to one side goes out walking straight, and astonished that his pain has gone. All I have done is to relieve the cramp in the big back muscles that has been causing the pain. As a follow-up I ask people who have improved in this way to keep on stretching their backs, using the floor of their bedrooms or living rooms as a substitute for my couch. Following up people like this in practice has been a joy. Over thirty years ago, I used the technique for a farmer who had been plagued with repeat acute back pain. He has not had an episode since, and whenever we meet he always reminds me of the day I 'stretched' him. I still wonder if that was much more due to luck on my part than real medical expertise.

However, there are drawbacks to manipulation. It is only of real use when the pain has been present for a relatively short time – say, less than a month. And it may cause damage, and cause more pain, if the problem is due to nerve root pressure. My own feeling is that all that most successful manipulation does is to stretch cramped back muscles. It is important here to stress the point about cramp yet again. Everyone knows what to do if they get cramp, for example, in a calf muscle. They pull up the foot, stretching the muscle, and the cramp, and the pain, disappear like magic. For cramp in the foot, they pull up the relevant toe, to do the same. I'm sure that all I do in stretching a back is to relieve a similar cramp. And once it has been relieved, the dysfunction is cured. It only needs to be done once. If it does not work first time, I am suspicious that there is something else wrong, and I do not attempt repeat manipulation.

As for long-term back pain, there is evidence, sadly, that manipulation may do more harm than good. Even enthusiastic medical manipulators warn against it in their textbooks, in case it causes permanent damage to the nerves in and emerging from the spine. My own tragic case of such damage, described in a previous chapter, in which a woman was paralysed for life by a manipulator, is a case in point.

However, it would be wrong to use her case as a warning against all manipulation. It happened in the late 1960s and is very unlikely to happen in today's climate of much closer professional regulation of manipulators. Today's doctors, thankfully, are allowed to meet professionally with osteopaths and chiropractors, and discuss patients' needs with them. Until the 1970s we could be struck off the medical register if we 'associated with such unqualified practitioners'. But it still stands as a warning. If you have a long-standing pain in the back, be very sure that you know its cause, and preferably see your doctor first, before visiting anyone without medical training who wants to use manipulation to treat you.

Exercise

I have been 'banging on' throughout this book about the need to exercise away back pain, and I make no apology about doing it again, in a bit more detail. First of all, the exercise must be started soon after the pain begins. Reputable trials of techniques to reduce back pain have proved that it is best started within the first two weeks, and even in the first few days if the pain is of the 'simple' type. Even if there is evidence of nerve root pain (see page 3), it helps to start exercise after a week or so.

Exercise isn't easy; it hurts at first. But because it is hurting, it does not mean it is harming. It should be aerobic, so walking, swimming and cycling (on a static bicycle) are good, and each period of exercise should be lengthy, more of an endurance test than a sprint. With each passing day, the duration of the exercise should be extended according to a timetable, to train the muscles. Walking, swimming and cycling are chosen because they put little strain on the back muscles: jogging and running may jar the back too much in the early stages of recovery. Weight training and exercises needing power should be avoided initially, as they may tear bruised muscles further.

The most important thing about the exercise is that you choose the exercise you enjoy most (or, if you hate all exercise, the one you loathe least). Two weeks after the start of the back pain, take advice, from someone suitably qualified to give it, about exercises to strengthen the tummy and back muscles. My own choice is a physiotherapist. Physiotherapy has developed along with sports medicine into a speciality of great skill and knowledge about muscles and their problems. We only have to see the miracles physiotherapists perform on the football field or at Wimbledon to see how they have progressed.

Note that today's physiotherapists will concentrate on active exercise – that is, something you will do yourself, and not something that the physiotherapist will do to you. It is not helpful to lie back and let someone else do the work: curing your back pain is almost entirely your own responsibility.

If your pain is not responding

If these fairly simple methods of treatment are not working, what can you do next? You have plenty of choice. Many different ways of treating back pain are put forward as effective, despite little scientific evidence to prove that they make any difference to the normal course of acute back pain.

They include injections into 'trigger points', and into joints and the epidural space (around the spinal cord). Some doctors swear *by* them; some swear *at* them. I am not convinced myself that they help, and they can have worrying, though thankfully rare, after-effects, such as infection or nerve or joint damage if not given with consummate accuracy. Probably the most positive evidence relates to epidural injections of steroids and local anaesthetics in people with true sciatica. Even so, there is a small risk of complications from such injections, and the potential benefit must be weighed against the possible risk. I do not lightly recommend an epidural for a case of back pain, and would refer the patient to a specialist, preferably in orthopaedics or in anaesthetics, to give it.

Acupuncture is rising in popularity for many conditions, most of them ill-defined, and back pain is one of them. I know of no scientific evidence to prove that acupuncture helps people with back pain more than a placebo would.

Instant pain relief can be achieved with ice, cold compresses, hot water bottles, heat lamps, short wave or ultrasound, or massage. What is used depends largely on the experience and preference of the physiotherapist treating you, or what you are most comfortable with. These methods may help for a while, but there is no proof that they shorten the course of the usual back-pain episode.

Putting people on traction (stretching the spine as on a rack) has gained favour recently, and if people have back muscle spasms, it seems to help a lot at the time. In many of them, however, the effect is short-lived and, like the treatments mentioned above, traction has not been proved to shorten significantly the duration of the back pain.

TENS (transcutaneous electrical nerve stimulation), a machine that transmits tiny electrical pulses into the area of the pain, has also been found wanting in clinical trials in back pain, although some patients (not in trials) report that they are helped by it.

Corrective equipment such as corsets to keep the back straight, and insoles fitted into shoes (in people whose back pain is put down to different lengths of leg), enjoyed their peak in popularity a decade or more ago. We hear little of them now. The corsets simply left the back muscles weaker and did not make a substantial difference to the pain. There is no real evidence that having one leg marginally shorter than the other (and therefore forcing the spine into a sideways-bent position) causes much back pain. The difference has to be around an inch or more before it is likely to affect the spine, and in most cases this has been noted and dealt with (by altering footwear) years before. As mentioned earlier, a short leg measurement (it is taken between the inside of the ankle to the projection of the pelvis above the hip, anatomically called the anterior superior ischial spine, or popularly the 'love handle') may well mean a crumbling hip joint. The treatment then is a replacement hip, rather than attention to the back.

Swedish researchers have found that bringing groups of back-pain sufferers together for education sessions about their pain has helped, particularly in workplaces, but it would be good to see the work repeated in Britain. Do the British respond in the same way? We don't yet know.

Treatments you should refuse

There are treatments for back pain that are not only ineffective, but can actually harm you. For example, if you need to have strong painkillers of the morphine type, such as morphine and high doses of codeine, for more than the first two weeks, then you need to be seen by a specialist and have further investigations. All these drugs are powerful promoters of addiction and lifelong dependency when given for pain, and the rules are very clear on how they should be used and for what. Long-term back pain is not one of the indications for them. The same goes for benzodiazepines, such as diazepam (Valium). If you continue to take diazepam for more than the first two weeks of your pain, you run a very high risk of becoming dependent upon it. Its long-term use can make you drowsy and mentally sluggish – absolutely not the state of mind you need for getting back to your normal working and social life.

Daily cortisone-like pills, such as prednisolone and triamcinolone, are drugs in the class of 'corticosteroids'. They may help in the short term if you have an inflammatory disease of the muscles and joints, but in the long term their use weakens bone by promoting the loss of calcium. In other words, they accelerate the degenerative process of osteoporosis, and instead of the backache easing as you grow older, it is likely to change in character and get worse.

Traction with bed rest may be comforting for the first few days, but is simply not effective in the long term. All it does is add stiffness, muscle wasting, loss of bone calcium, pressure sores, and even deep vein thrombosis to your troubles. The same goes for being put in plaster jackets, which can also cause breathing problems. At the risk of being repetitive, it must be stressed again that you must be active, and not passive, in your fight against your back pain.

Although manipulation is recommended in the acute stage (see page 44), you must refuse any suggestion that your back be manipulated under anaesthetic. This was a popular treatment in the early 1990s, until Haldeman and Rubinstein highlighted its dangers in 1992 (Haldeman and Rubinstein, 1992, pp. 1469–73). They showed that it could cause serious damage to the nerves in the base of the spine, leaving some people with severe and permanent difficulties in controlling their ability to pass urine and open their bowels. If you are to be manipulated it is vital you remain conscious throughout, so that you can tell the manipulator when you are in pain.

8
Reconditioning your back (2) – what you can do yourself

When people with back pain are asked what they want to know most about their pain, there are four points that crop up again and again. They wish to know:

- How long they will have the pain and the physical limitations it will put upon them.
- How to manage their pain most effectively.
- How they can get quickly back to their normal activities.
- How to prevent and minimize the severity of any future episodes.

Recognizing these concerns, medical authorities in countries like the United States, Britain, Germany and New Zealand have issued guidelines to doctors on how to give their patients up-to-date and accurate information on their problems. What is unique about the British approach is that our 'Back Book' is not written with a medical slant. Quite rightly, it makes back pain almost a normal aspect of life, something that anyone can have, and not an illness experienced by a 'sick' minority.

The Back Book is very inexpensive and can be bought from the Stationery Office, St Crispins, Duke Street, Norwich NR3 1PD, or from most good bookshops (ISBN 0-11-702078-8). It is well worth buying for anyone with back pain. It gives advice on how to deal with your own backache, how to recover as quickly as possible, how to stay active and avoid long-term disability, and how to return to a normal life.

What follows here are a few practical points from *The Back Book* about acute back pain.

The book emphasizes that back pain is not usually due to serious disease, and that most attacks settle quickly; it need not disable you unless you let it. It stresses that activity, rather than rest, is best from the start: that the back is designed for movement, and that when it is kept moving you feel better. The people who cope best with back pain are those who stay active and get on with their lives in spite of their pain.

The spine is exceptionally strong, with a column of solid bony cylinders, kept together by strong muscles and ligaments, between which are rubber-like discs to give it strength, flexibility and stability. It is very difficult to damage the spine with normal use. So most people with back pain have no spinal problems, nor have they 'slipped discs' or 'trapped nerves'. Even if they do have a slipped disc it usually cures itself. X-ray findings of 'degeneration' in the lower spine are normal in older people, much like wrinkles in the skin or grey hair. They do not signify arthritis or serious spinal disease and they cannot be linked with back pain.

The Back Book then stresses that in most people the exact source of the pain cannot be identified, and that can be frustrating. But that can also be looked on as good news, rather than bad, because any serious disease or injury has been ruled out. Your back is just 'out of condition' and the answer is to get it working properly again. Stress plays its part in this: it can cause muscle tension and cramp, and directly causes pain. So dealing with the stress and exercising are the two main lines of attack upon your pain.

I have dealt in general on the exercises that will help, such as walking, cycling and swimming. Of course, when you are in pain it isn't easy to force yourself to do these things. But there are specific hints on what to do and what to avoid, thus making it easier to exercise.

First, here are the 'do's':

- When lifting, know your limits – what you can handle and what you can't. Always keep the object you are lifting close to your body, preferably near your navel. Lift by bending your knees, not your back, and use your leg muscles to lift and lower the weight. Never rotate your spine while carrying a weight. If you must turn while holding a weight – say, lifting from the floor or a workbench and then turning a right angle to load a car or van – then keep straight and turn your whole body round with your feet. Always keep your toes pointing in the same direction as your nose.
- When sitting, use a chair with a hard, straight, vertical back. Put a slim cushion in the small of your back (a folded towel will do). Rise from the chair and walk around every half an hour or so.
- When standing, you may feel more comfortable with one foot on a low stool. That's why bars in pubs etc. have foot rails along

them, so that people can lean at the bar with one leg bent. Years ago, someone designing bars must have had a sore back prior to coming up with this idea! If you have to stand at work, your work surface must be at the right height for you.

- When driving, move the seat until your legs are at the right distance from the pedals, and your body and legs are in the same plane. Do not drive for long periods with your legs pointing off to one side from your hips. If the car pedals do not allow you to sit with your stomach and your legs facing in the same direction, drive a car with controls that do. As with sitting in a chair, if you can organize support to the small of your back, do so. It may be by adjusting the cushioning inside the back of the seat: if your seat doesn't allow that, then that folded towel may come in useful.

- When walking, cycling or swimming, make time for at least 30–40 minutes of brisk exercise every day. Then increase it day by day.

- When sleeping, use a firm mattress. Some people recommend a hard mattress, or even putting the mattress on the floor or on boards. The evidence that a hard mattress is better than a firm one isn't great. The important thing is not to sleep on too soft a mattress, as you may well wake in the morning with stiff and painful muscles.

- Try to relax. There are many methods by which you can relax your muscles, including yoga, transcendental meditation and the Alexander technique. They all combine ways of controlling your breathing, calming your mind, and improving your muscle tone. There is more about them in Chapter 10. Here it is enough to state that relaxing muscles helps to relieve pain.

Now come the 'don'ts':

- Never lift or carry something without thinking first about how heavy it is and how you are going to do it. I have only once had acute back pain, and it was after carrying several boxes of office paper to my car, a distance of about a quarter of a mile. It was a heavy load, and by the time I got to the boot of my car I didn't want to put it down and then lift it into the car. So I swung it into the open boot, with my feet static. Instantly I knew I had hurt my back. It was a full month before I was completely pain-free again. It was an idiotic thing to do, and I'm supposed to know something about how to care for my back!

- Don't sit on a soft easy chair with a low seat and no real back support. And do not sit for hours in one position.
- The same goes for standing. Do not stand for a long time in one position. If you are standing for a lengthy period in one position at work, ask to vary your position and have a seat provided that takes the weight off your back muscles. Any good employer would rather do that than have you off work – and that can be the alternative.
- Don't drive for hours without a break, and plan your stops at hourly intervals. They don't need to be long – just a walk and stretch round the car will do.
- As for exercise, don't become a couch potato. Sitting around all day, no matter how comfortable the couch, will eventually get to your back by weakening and stiffening your muscles. If you must watch a favourite programme, put the exercise bike in front of the TV and start pedalling as you watch. Then you can get the best of both worlds.
- Sleeping is all very well. We all need to have around five to six hours' sleep each night as a minimum, but staying in bed too long is a big mistake. That, too, stiffens and weakens your back muscles. Get up early each morning and you will have time to do a little exercise before breakfast. There are plenty of 'morning stretching programmes' on TV to which you can limber up.
- And don't worry or become tense and anxious, for that will heighten the pain. If you find yourself tensing up, actively seek relaxation. One of the programmes described in the next chapter may suit you.

The Back Book also explains what doctors can do – and what they can't.

There is the old story about the doctor who was asked to cure a cold. He told his patient to go and lie naked in the cold and rain. His patient was astonished by this advice, and asked why he had to do this. His doctor replied, 'Well, if you do that, you will get pneumonia. I can cure pneumonia, but I can't cure your cold.'

Acute backache is something like that. It's like the common cold – a minor, though very inconvenient and uncomfortable, problem that will pass. When doctors are faced with the rare patient who does have a serious back disease (the analogy is the pneumonia), they can make a passable attempt at curing most of them. But they can do little with simple back pain. They can help you over the first few days of pain, but the biggest effort has to come from you.

There are a few warning signs that tell you that you must see your doctor urgently. They include:

- pain that is getting worse, rather than better, as the days go by;
- any difficulty in being able to pass urine or in controlling its flow;
- numbness (loss of the feeling of touch and/or pinprick) around the anus or genital area, or in the skin in between them, the perineum;
- numbness, pins and needles (the medical term is paraesthesia) and/or weakness in both legs;
- loss of balance or difficulty in keeping steady.

These are all signs that there is pressure on the centre of the lowest section of the spinal cord, and that something must be done immediately to relieve it. You may need urgent decompressing surgery. However, this is very rare. In my career as a doctor, which goes back to the 1960s, I have only come across two such cases: one being in a major hospital, and the other occurring many years ago in general practice. So keep in mind my recurring theme throughout this book: that your pain very rarely has a serious cause that needs emergency treatment in hospital.

So now you know about back pain, what next matters is your own attitude to it. *The Back Book* describes two main reactions to pain. It divides people into 'avoiders' and 'copers'. What happens to you in the long term very much depends upon the group in which you slot yourself.

Avoiders are frightened by their pain and worry about what is to happen to them. The tension makes their pain worse. Avoiders also equate pain with damage, so they avoid anything that might provoke it. They therefore rest, and wait for the pain to lessen. When it doesn't, they worry further, become more tense, and the pain worsens. They suffer far more than copers. Their pain lasts longer, they have more time away from their work, and they often become chronically disabled by their pain and their mental reaction to it.

Copers accept that the pain will improve and that they do not need to fear the future. They continue with their daily routine as far as they can. They have a positive attitude and remain energetic and at work. Their pain fades faster than that of the avoiders, and they are generally healthier over the years to come.

Obviously it is far better to be a coper than an avoider. I quote here again from *The Back Book*, showing you how to become a coper:

- Keep up as many of your daily activities as possible. Avoid heavy lifting and heaving, but that's all.
- Keep yourself fit with your favourite exercise. Exercising your back will make you feel better.
- Do a bit more every day, and take pleasure in measuring your progress. It will stimulate you to do more still, and get you back to normality sooner.
- Stay at work. If you normally do heavy work, ask for light work for two weeks or so.
- Accept the odd setback. From time to time, your back will complain for a while with the odd spasm, sharp twinge or dull ache. They do not mean you are going backwards. Patients are well named, especially if they have backache. The one quality they need above all others is patience.
- Don't become dependent on drugs to kill the pain. They are all right for the first few days but, after that, use exercise and relaxation to fight it.
- Don't stay in, nursing your pain and misery: force yourself to go out and enjoy yourself. If you get a spasm when you are out, try to laugh at it. It isn't easy, but it works.
- Don't worry. If you have simple back pain you will not become an invalid. It will get better, completely.
- Above all, don't heed other people's stories about bad backs. They are invariably exaggerated, and often relate to people at third or fourth hand. These tales grow like Chinese whispers as they are passed on from person to person.
- Don't get depressed on a bad day. It really will get better.
- Finally, you have to live your life. You need to do what you want to do. Don't let your 'bad back' spoil that.

9

Osteopathy, chiropractic and physiotherapy

No book on back pain would be complete without a chapter on osteopathy, chiropractic and physiotherapy. An Australian friend tells me that no one there with back pain would dream of initially consulting a medical doctor with it. They would visit an osteopath instead. Of course, this may be related to the Australian health care system, in which you have to pay a doctor or an osteopath equally for consultations and treatments. In Britain, medical practitioners are free, and osteopaths are not. So most people go to their GPs. But it has to be accepted that osteopaths have acquired a reputation for treating back pain – and that GPs have not.

Osteopathy, chiropractic and physiotherapy are all approaches to the treatment of back pain. They developed out of the feeling that if there is pain in the back, something mechanical, or physical, must be wrong with it. The corollary to that belief, of course, is that if the trouble is truly mechanical, then the treatment should also be mechanical. A mechanical problem should have a mechanical solution.

Having read this far, you should now be convinced that back pain and its treatment are not as simple as that. To be fair to the proponents of osteopathy and chiropractic, however, their views should be included here.

To put osteopathy and chiropractic into a modern perspective, we need to know something of their history. It is a long and venerable, though controversial, one. There have been manipulators for hundreds of years. Hippocrates described manipulation of the spine more than two thousand years ago. In places as distant as Norway and Mexico, medicine men trampled spines to relieve back pain. In medieval Europe, there were bone-setter families who passed on their knowledge from father to son for generations. Relations between bone setters and orthodox doctors varied from a wary respect to downright hostility.

By the nineteenth century the battle lines were drawn. The speciality of orthopaedic surgery had emerged from the military surgeons and the academic surgeons dealing with wounds, accidents and bone disease. Manipulations remained acceptable for treating fractures, but they were rejected for straightforward back pain. For that, the surgeons recommended rest, and if that did not work, immobilization – in effect, creating more disability rather than less.

Not only did the medical profession turn against manipulation, it forbade doctors from even associating with unqualified persons who practised manipulation. Doctors like myself, when we were students, were told about the five 'A's' that would get us struck off the medical register if we indulged in them. They were Adultery (with a patient), Advertising (for patients), Alcoholism, Addiction (to drugs), and Associating with unqualified practitioners. This last was at least as heinous as all the others, and was directly aimed at osteopaths and chiropractors.

The medical profession of the nineteenth and twentieth centuries had only itself to blame for the rise in the popularity of those whom they perceived as enemies. One reason was doctors' lack of success with their 'rest and your body will heal itself' approach. Few people were patient enough to follow this advice, and in any case it was manifestly unsuccessful. Because of this, orthodox practitioners earned the reputation of being uninterested in back pain – and the successors of the bone setters reaped the benefits.

The medical scene in the latter half of the nineteenth century was therefore a perfect time for the rise of osteopathy and chiropractic – they offered active remedies for aches and pains, and opportunities for people to shake them off, and return sooner to normal life and work.

It may now be useful to look at some of the differences in these various techniques.

Osteopathy

Osteopathy arrived first, as the brainchild of Dr Andrew Still. Writing in 1899 (Still, 1899), he tells of his launch of the new branch of medicine in 1874. A practising doctor himself, he turned against orthodox medicine when it could not prevent the deaths of three of his children from meningitis. He turned against drugs, too, because his brother had become addicted to morphine after its prescription by a colleague. He therefore turned back to what he believed were the principles of the father of medicine, Hippocrates, more than two thousand years before.

In the 1870s this was entirely understandable, as few of the medicines prescribed then were beneficial, and many were dangerous and even poisonous. Patients of Still's time were more likely to be made more ill, rather than less, by visiting their doctors.

Here are Still's two main principles by which he practised from 1874 onwards. They remain the mainstay of the philosophy of osteopathy today:

1 The body has in itself the power to combat disease, and we should not interfere with this power, as this will hinder Nature's attempt towards recovery.
2 We humans are machines subject to the same mechanical principles and failures as a steam engine. The cause of disease is 'dislocated' bones, disorders of ligaments and cramped muscles, especially in the back, putting pressure on the circulation and nerves. This leads to ischaemia (lack of blood supply to the relevant tissues) and necrosis (death of tissues), partly due to blocking of the life force travelling along nerves. This Dr Still called the osteopathic lesion – hence the name for his system of healing.

He believed that osteopathy, by relocating bones, easing the ligament problems and relaxing the muscles, would allow the body's defences to heal the underlying ailment.

Of course, as we have learned more about the human body, Still's ideas on ischaemia, necrosis and the life force have been updated. Still believed that manipulation did not cure problems, but put the body's structure in such a position that any 'lesion' was more amenable to the body's self-healing powers.

By the 1990s, osteopaths were explaining that their system was based on the belief that a body with a normal mechanical structure that is well nourished will mount its own defences against most diseases. Although osteopathy is mostly used to treat symptoms such as pain, its main principle is still to achieve 'normal body mechanics' because they are held to be central to good health (DiGiovanna and Schiowitz, 1991). Osteopaths believe that if they can correct problems in the nerves, muscles and skeleton they will help the body to heal itself of most diseases, even if they seem quite apart from and distant from the spine. They see the body as an integrated whole, able to heal itself given the best circumstances, which the osteopath does his or her best to create with manipulation.

The modern osteopath comes to a diagnosis of what is wrong in the back on three criteria, defined as ART by leading osteopaths E. L. DiGiovanna and S. Schiowitz (DiGiovanna and Schiowitz, 1991). A is for asymmetry, in which one vertebra may lie slightly 'off-line', i.e. asymmetrically in relation to the other vertebrae. R is for restricted movement, which may be stiffer than normal, causing pain or becoming limited in comparison to normal. The restriction is thought to be caused by some problem in a bone, a joint or a tendon, and this can be relieved by manipulation. T is for tissue changes, that can be felt by the osteopath on examining the skin, tissues or muscles next to an affected joint.

Most osteopaths have abandoned the idea that joints in the spinal column may actually be 'out of place', as there is no evidence that this can happen in normal life. Anyone who has studied the human spine quickly realizes that it would take tremendous force to dislocate any joint between two vertebrae in the back, especially when they are surrounded by the mass of muscles and powerful ligaments in a normally healthy human.

There is also little evidence that people with back pain are restricted in their movements. Studies by our old friend Professor Waddell and by A. K. Burton and colleagues (Burton and colleagues, 1990, pp. 262–8) have shown that people with back pain can flex their backs just as far as those with no pain. Sufferers of back pain are as likely to have over-mobile as under mobile backs – or backs that are normally flexible.

As for changes in the texture of the tissues, osteopaths have described them as thickening or thinning, dry or 'boggy', rough or smooth, board-like or stringy, tender or not, red or pale. Muscles may be bulky with regular use, or wasted with lack of use. It is difficult to relate these changes consistently with any particular type of pain, and the appearances and 'feel' of the skin and underlying tissues may even change in any one person from day to day.

So it is not easy for doctors like myself, who are untrained in the details of osteopathic examination, to pass judgement on it. All I can add is that whether or not the theory of osteopathy passes scientific scrutiny, some people with back pain obviously benefit from it in practice.

This has been recognized for many years in the United States. In 1968, the American Medical Association stopped its opposition to osteopathy, so that today, being a doctor of osteopathy (a graduate of one of the 15 American colleges of osteopathy) in the United States is the equivalent of being a doctor of medicine. Although the British School of Osteopathy was established in 1917, the first Act of Parliament to register and oversee osteopaths had to wait until 1993. It is only since then that orthodox doctors have been officially allowed to refer patients to them and, even now, very few patients are offered osteopathic treatment within the NHS. The numbers are growing, though.

I am not against osteopathy. Because I have seen good, and even sometimes spectacular, results from my small experience of manipulation, I am happy to accept that osteopathic manipulation will help some people. Osteopaths, by their training, obviously have much more experience than me in manipulating spinal muscles. However, I do have serious doubts when patients tell me that they have to have a series of treatments over several weeks. In my experience, if manipulation is going to work, it does so at the first attempt. I believe that is because the pain is caused by cramp in the large back muscles, and stretching them relieves the cramp, and therefore the pain. If that does not happen, repeated attempts to cure the pain will fail.

I also do not subscribe to the theory that if you get the posture correct by manipulation, your body will heal itself of the pain. There are many more causes of pain than a wrong posture, and many more ways of helping healing than to leave the body's defences to help themselves. We are in the twenty-first century now, and not stuck in the nineteenth. We have penicillin and vaccines now to cure and prevent meningitis, and we have many effective painkillers that have allowed doctors to abandon their nineteenth-century dependence on morphine. I wonder if Dr Still would have invented osteopathy if he had had these weapons in his armoury against disease.

Chiropractic

The man who founded chiropractic, D. D. Palmer, was not a doctor but a magnetic healer. He began the first chiropractic clinic in Iowa, in 1895. Although there are some similarities between chiropractic and osteopathy, Palmer held widely different views from Dr Still.

Palmer believed that most back pain was caused by what he termed 'subluxations' of various vertebrae. These are slight malpositions of a vertebra in its relationship to the one above or below it.

According to Palmer, these caused pressures on nerves (he did not believe they harmed the blood flow through the spinal area), and that this pressure was what caused the pain. He claimed to be 'the first to replace displaced vertebrae by using the spinous or transverse processes (of the vertebrae) as levers, whereby to rack (them) into normal position' (Palmer, 1910).

This was not all. Palmer laid much emphasis on 'vitalism'. This is the life force, the fundamental ability of the body to heal itself. He believed that illness was due to the person's lowered resistance to disease, and that only by building up that resistance could the person be healed. So chiropractic stresses the need for a good diet, a healthy lifestyle and good surroundings in which to live. It avoids drugs and surgery, and impresses on patients that their illness is caused by their failure to maintain their health. Chiropractic healing depends a lot on the doctor-patient relationship and the confidence that grows between the two. It is as far from the prescription-happy GP as it is possible to be. Chiropractic claims that it heals the whole person, rather than trying to cure a specific disease.

I have some problems with this approach. My main one is that if patients do not get relief from their pain, they may well feel guilty about it. They blame themselves, wrongly, for falling short of their chiropractor's ideal, and this is something to be deplored. There are times when orthodox medical treatment and surgery must be considered, and it is incumbent on chiropractors to remember this.

Happily, most modern chiropractors accept that they must combine their holistic approach with referral to their medical colleagues when it is needed. So I am not against chiropractic, provided that the patient benefits almost immediately. I have the same reservation about chiropractic as I have about osteopathy. If the chiropractor is unable to ease the pain at the first visit, it is unlikely to be eased by further manipulations. I am also uneasy about the use of X-rays by chiropractors to make their diagnoses. As mentioned elsewhere in this book, X-ray appearances do not readily correlate with the presence or extent of back pain. And taking clear X-rays of the back means high radiation doses. If you do not need an X-ray you should not have one. And certainly you should not submit yourself to repeated X-rays.

As with osteopathy, I must admit to scepticism about chiropractors' belief that 'subluxations' of spinal joints exist and cause pain. I am even more sceptical that simply by using one's fingers and hands one can reduce these subluxations. And when I hear, as I did in October 2002, that there are chiropractors who can manipulate the spines of horses, I am lost in admiration for their abilities.

Today, chiropractic is now recognized as a respectable speciality by the medical world. Like osteopaths, chiropractors had to wait a long time in Britain before they were accepted. The Anglo-European College of Chiropractic (the first British training institution for the speciality) started in 1965, and the Act regulating chiropractic was passed by Parliament in 1994. So if you wish to see a chiropractor, your GP is allowed to refer you to one. However, you are more likely to be referred to a physiotherapist, who will probably work within the NHS.

Physiotherapy

Physiotherapy has always enjoyed respectability: unlike osteopathy and chiropractic, it did not have to fight for it. It started in Britain in 1894, as a Society of Trained Masseuses. By 1920, when the Society was given its Royal Charter, it trained people in massage, medical gymnastics, electrotherapies and similar treatment methods. American physiotherapy grew out of the need to rehabilitate soldiers returning from the First World War, so it put more emphasis on exercise and on minimizing disabilities than on massage.

The modern physiotherapist is an independent expert in the health care team, who examines patients with physical problems to make a diagnosis and determine treatments. These treatments include exercise, mobilization and manipulation, the use of electrical and other modes of treatment (such as ultrasound and heat), and training in self-help in the home and for return to normal life and work. Physiotherapists are also expert in the equipment needed for help if you have a disability, and in promoting fitness and guidance on how to attain a better quality of life.

So when you are referred to a physiotherapist you can expect much more than just attention for a short while to your back pain. You and your 'physio' will spend considerable time discussing what you can do, not just to ease your pain, but to change all aspects of your life so that it will not return or become worse.

In the United Kingdom, most general practice teams now have an attached physiotherapist to whom their patients with back pain are referred. In my own experience of eight or more practices in the south-west of Scotland, physiotherapists are a huge asset, who are not only expert at relieving acute pain, but have the time to discuss with each patient all the aspects of their problems that need to be aired. It is not for them simply a matter of manipulation, although that obviously can play a part. At practice team case conferences, physiotherapists often provide the clues to diagnosis and treatment that have been missed by the doctors.

Of course, physiotherapists are professionals who practise in their own right, independently of the primary care teams. In Britain, they should be members of the Chartered Society of Physiotherapy. If you are thinking of seeing one privately, it is a courtesy to let your doctor know you are doing so, and to give the physiotherapist your doctor's name and address. There should be full co-operation between them.

10
Relaxing

Because a main theme of this book has been that people with back pain should actively exercise, rather than rest, it doesn't follow that you shouldn't take time to relax. Relaxation is not an alternative to exercise, but is complementary to it. How you relax, however, can make a big difference.

People promote several systems to help people relax. Yoga is one, transcendental meditation another, the Alexander technique yet another. They are all effective in their own way, and you will want to choose the one that suits your personality and helps your pain most. The main benefit from them is that they improve your posture. When standing or sitting, or even lying down, many of us tense the muscles that lie around our spines (from neck to pelvis). Our spines are a little twisted, and the discordance between one set of muscles and another initiates the spasm that leads to backache. The most common form of bad posture is a rounded upper back – a 'hump', with head jutting forward, neck at an angle, and shoulders hunched and cramped.

Relaxation, no matter which method you use, loosens all the tension, and eases the pain accordingly. I admit to finding the simplest method the best. To relax all the spinal muscles, just lie on your back on the floor. A thick book, like a dictionary, is the only prop you need. Put it under the back of your head, so that the head is not arched back, but almost straight on your neck. The chin should feel very slightly tucked in, but it mustn't be anywhere near to being down on your chest. Have the feeling that you have slightly stretched your neck to get it to rest on the book.

Now lie there, with arms outstretched sideways and hands relaxed (slightly curled fingers) for a full ten minutes. Shut your eyes, and listen to whatever music you like best on the radio or by playing a CD or cassette. While you are lying there, go from head to toe in your mind, relaxing each group of muscles in turn. Start with the scalp, then the face, the neck, the shoulders, the upper arms, the forearms, the hands, and the fingers. Now turn to the upper trunk, back and front, the waist muscles, the lower back and stomach muscles, the groins and hips. Finally, loosen the muscles of the thighs, shins, calves, feet and toes. Don't miss any of them.

As you are doing this, you will find that you are naturally stretching your body and limbs, so that your feet are an inch or two further from your head than when you started. That may impress on you how tense your muscles have been.

After that first ten minutes, you can now stretch your spine and limbs further. Still lying on your back, swing your right arm upwards and backwards so that it is reaching out horizontally, along the carpet in the same line as your body. If you were standing you would now be reaching upwards to the roof. Now stretch the arm as far along that line as you can, while at the same time stretching your right leg down to the tips of your toes, as far as you can. Hold that for a few seconds, then relax. Do the same for the left arm and leg. Rest for a few minutes, then repeat the exercise, and repeat it once or twice more. Then relax your whole body again for another ten minutes before getting up. Get up by rolling over on to one side, then gently rising from one knee, keeping the small of the back hollow as you do so.

The whole exercise should take only 25 minutes, or 30 minutes at the most. If you can take time to do that every day, you should feel some benefit. I'm afraid my evidence for this is only anecdotal. I have no clinical trial results to back it up, but it does seem to work for many of my back-pain patients.

Alexander technique

The exercise above is taken (and modified slightly) from the Alexander technique. Matthias Alexander was not a doctor. He was an Australian actor and theatre director, born in 1870, who came to fame in the 1930s. To be honest, even his friends and relatives admitted he was a 'rogue' (Barlow, 1986). He was a showman, and travelled around promoting his method as giving people perfect health. As he was unqualified in medicine, his outrageous claims naturally upset the establishment, so the Alexander techniques were for many years outside the mainstream of medical thought.

But he had a point. Being an actor, rather than a doctor, he was naturally interested in posture. He proposed that many of people's ills were due to muscle tension that pulled the spine out of shape. Aches and pains, he suggested, could be cured by getting one's posture right. The head had to be held square, the shoulders open, the neck vertical, the spine straight, the lower back neither too hollow nor too bowed, the knees straight. The body had not to be allowed to sag or to be too tense.

Today his more exaggerated claims are laughable, but his thoughts on backache and posture are still valid. The exercise I have described, of lying on one's back on the floor, and letting the spine, from neck to the lower back, stretch and straighten with gravity, certainly helps a lot of people. If you would like to read more about him and his methods, Wilfred Barlow's book, *The Alexander Principle*, may still be found in libraries. There are Alexander practitioners, mostly physiotherapists and nurses, in most districts: they should be in your local telephone directory. They should hold the certificate of the Society of Teachers of the Alexander Technique (STAT) if they are genuine.

11

When the pain has become 'chronic'

Every doctor who treats people with acute back pain has one overriding aim in mind – to prevent it from becoming 'chronic'. By this is not meant a back pain that comes and goes over many months. That is recurrent acute pain, and is dealt with in the ways described in the previous chapters.

Chronic pain is something different. It is the pain that is nagging away, virtually all the time. It keeps people off work for months and even years. It often causes them to lose their jobs. Their quality of life has been devastated by their back problem. They believe that their problems would disappear if only their back pain could be cured. They ask for more and more appointments to specialists, including neurosurgeons and orthopaedic surgeons. And at the end of all the investigations, including sometimes drastic surgery, they are still left with their chronic back pain.

Does this sound familiar? I presume, because you have read this far, there is a high chance that you or someone you care for are in this category. And obviously you are desperate to find in these pages an answer.

Bear with me, because what follows isn't comforting reading. In researching all the methods that have become popular for the treatment of back pain, very few have stood up to scrutiny. We do not have a good, fast, easy medical or surgical solution to chronic back pain. But we may have other approaches that will help.

Let's take the usual approaches first – those that we considered for acute back pain:

- *Painkilling drugs*: Aspirin-like drugs such as ibuprofen, naproxen, indomethacin, and aspirin itself, do give short-term relief from pain. But they are not a long-term answer. As the effects of the drugs wear off, the pain returns, and the next dose has to be taken. Many people with chronic back pain are on the maximum doses of anti-inflammatory and analgesic drugs every day of their lives. In the long term this cannot be good for them, especially as their effectiveness wears off. At the same time, these drugs' potential for causing unwanted effects, such as stomach ulcers, increases.

- *Antidepressant drugs*: Antidepressant drugs help ease the pain of nerve root pressure. They also help, naturally, as this is why they were developed, to lift the mood of people who are depressed. Not surprisingly, this is a fairly high proportion of people with chronic pain. There are dozens of antidepressants, but, as mentioned earlier in the book, most fall into two main groups – the 'tricyclics' and the 'selective serotonin reuptake inhibitors' (SSRIs). If you need them, your doctor will discuss with you which of them will be suitable and their possible side effects.

- *Injections*: For the very few people whose chronic back pain is caused by disc pressure on a nerve root, injections of either local anaesthetic or steroid (such as hydrocortisone) into the site gives short-term relief. There does not seem to be any advantage of one type of injection over the other. However, such injections do nothing for the vast majority of people with chronic low back pain.

- *Manipulation*: There is good evidence that manipulation (strangely, the type of manipulation does not seem to matter) helps chronic back pain. By good evidence is meant a 1996 survey of no less than 80 trials of 14 different types of treatment of chronic low back pain, reported by Dr van Tulder and his colleagues (van Tulder and colleagues, 1996, pp. 245–95). They concluded that manipulation was considerably more effective in easing pain than giving placebos, and moderately more effective than most other treatments.

- *Traction*: Only one small trial is reported on the value of traction for chronic pain: it was not shown to be effective either in reducing pain or improving disability.

- *TENS*: TENS machines are popular, but sadly there is little evidence that they help to ease long-term backache. Like other treatments for pain, they can help in the short term, and give welcome relief in episodes of acute back pain. But the trials show that they do not have a long-term effect on chronic pain.

- *Acupuncture*: The difficulty with assessing trials of acupuncture is that it is almost impossible to construct a study in which the results can be subjected to independent statistical analysis without bias. Although there are six well-conducted scientific trials comparing acupuncture with other treatments and/or sham acupuncture, they give contradictory results. The jury must still be considered to be in doubt about the effects of acupuncture in chronic back pain. My own experience of people who tried acupuncture is that it failed to make any difference, but I confess I am not a fan, so I may be biased against it.

- *Exercise*: There is no doubt that exercise helps people with acute back pain to get better faster and to return to work earlier than those who rest. But does it do the same for chronic back pain? And does it matter what kind of exercise you do?

These questions concerning exercise have occupied the minds of many researchers. The first answer is clear: exercise helps. The three best-planned and analysed trials all showed that exercise helps to relieve chronic back pain and to ease people with it back towards a normal life (van Tulder and colleagues, 1996). However, the exercise must be fairly strenuous. Hansen and his colleagues have shown that to get significant improvement in the pain, patients need to learn to do intense, dynamic back exercises to control their pain and get their backs working again as they should (Hansen and colleagues, 1993, pp. 98–107).

Another team of researchers found that a full fitness programme was more effective at relieving the chronic pain than a programme of exercises performed at home (Frost and colleagues, 1992, pp. 151–4). However, the difficulty in all these reports is that a year after the treatments had started, most of the people in the studies still had their back pain. It seems, then, that we must do more than subject our patients to intensive exercise if we are to cure their pain.

So is there another approach? For more than thirty years now, the Scandinavians have had 'back schools' in which groups of people with chronic low back pain have been taught together to understand their problems and how to deal with them. They are given lessons on the structures in, and the working of, the back, in how to move at home and at work without putting it under strain. They are then encouraged to put the theory into practice by being given exercises to do. Such schools are multiplying throughout Europe and the United States. They seem less popular in Britain. Whether they have great success is difficult to say, because there are no reliable figures to show that such schools are more successful at getting people with chronic back pain back to work sooner than those who have not been to them.

To summarize: the numbers of different treatments, and their relatively poor results, suggest that the way we doctors treat back pain at the moment is not good enough. Could the psychologists do any better? Maybe they can.

12
Chronic pain – bringing in the brain

In the last two decades, hospitals all over Britain have set up 'Pain Clinics'. Staffed principally by anaesthetists with an interest in pain, but also by doctors from other disciplines, they deal with people with many different diseases but with one thing in common. They have incessant pain, and conventional treatments have failed them. The aim of the Pain Clinics is not to cure a disease (the patients' other specialists have that responsibility), but to help people manage their pain. Many of the people attending Pain Clinics have chronic low back pain – a measure of how ineffective we GPs and orthopaedic surgeons are in treating them.

So where are we going wrong? In the past, doctors looked on pain as merely a symptom of injury or disease, and focused on the causes of the pain, and how to treat them. But we know now that we cannot pinpoint the cause of most back pain. Even when we can, we still tend to treat pain as a physical symptom – something to treat with physical medications like drugs and electrical impulses like TENS machines. What we have forgotten is that pain is a *perception*, something that occurs in the brain. It is heightened by stress and anxiety, and it changes depending on the mood we are in. If that is the case, then ways of lowering our levels of pain may also depend on our mood and our mental approach to our pain. If we can improve these things, perhaps we can deal better with the pain. Although we may not know the precise cause of the pain, we may still use mental attitudes to diminish it or at least tolerate it better.

So the aim of the staff in Pain Clinics is not just to prescribe physical methods to ease pain, but to help people cope with their pain and manage it so that it does not harm their quality of life. That may sound a tall order if you are in pain now, but it is certainly a fresh approach that is worth trying.

Behavioural therapy

The first, and still a well-used, approach to treating pain in this way was called behavioural management (Fordyce, 1976). It is, at first sight, quite a cruel system, but it does work. Behavioural therapists observe their subjects who have chronic pain, and assess them for either 'pain behaviour' or 'well behaviour'. They then try to reinforce the well behaviour and to get the patient to abandon their pain behaviour. Examples of pain behaviour include limping, fidgeting, resting, taking painkilling drugs, seeking sympathy from friends, and avoiding social and work duties and contacts. Examples of well behaviour are physical activity and normal social interactions. People on behaviour pain-management regimes are told to take their drugs at prearranged fixed times during the day, not when they have pain. They are asked to exercise, too, at fixed times during the day.

It is crucial to the success of behavioural therapy that the staff at the clinic and the relatives and close friends of the sufferer co-operate fully in the treatment. So the family need to know how to reinforce the well behaviour and ignore the pain behaviour.

Behavioural therapy on its own can be very hard to keep up, especially for the family, who may be perceived as being unfeeling and unnecessarily cruel. So most pain experts combine it with the second approach – cognitive therapy.

Cognitive therapy

Modern theories on how pain arises and is perceived by the brain accept that thoughts and feelings can alter its intensity and duration. In cognitive therapy (cognitive simply means understanding) the therapist discusses the meaning of pain with the patient. The discussion ranges over fears and beliefs about pain, and how it can be dealt with, and the patient's expectations about the treatment. It then progresses to how the patient can develop their own expertise in dealing with their particular pain. In the process, the patient becomes more self-confident that the pain can be beaten by his or her own efforts.

In cognitive therapy people learn to avoid or stop dwelling on their pain – for example, by thinking of something else, or even changing their perception of pain into another feeling. If you think that is impossible, think of the experience of Odette Churchill, in the Second World War.

Odette was a British agent who was caught by the Nazis in occupied France. In writing my first book, *Human Potential, The*

Limits and Beyond, in 1980, my co-author, Wendy Cooper, and I had the privilege of interviewing Odette about her experience with the Gestapo. Brought to the interrogation room, she knew that she had to hold out for at least 24 hours to let her resistance colleagues get away. The Gestapo started to pull her fingernails out, one by one, using pliers. Despite the terrible pain, she drew down in front of her eyes an imaginary cinema screen, and on it played an imaginary home movie in which there were scenes of picnics with her husband and daughters in the English countryside. She was able to keep quiet for the required day, and none of her group were betrayed.

Odette only survived because of her surname: the Gestapo thought, wrongly, that she might have a family connection with Winston Churchill, and would have used her as a bargaining pawn if the war were to be lost. Which is how Wendy and I came to hear her remarkable story at first hand. She was a remarkable woman, but she was modest too. She believed strongly that anyone in a crisis could deal with pain as she did, by concentrating on something else. In fact, she was a perfect example of good cognitive therapy for pain.

I'm not sure that everyone has the mental powers of Odette, but, with help, we can go a long way along that path.

Cognitive therapy has two other aspects. Stress makes pain worse. Under cognitive therapy, people are taught how to deal better with stress, and to use their new knowledge when the pain returns or worsens. They are also taught how to practise and improve their ability to manage pain and stress, being especially aware of conditions that may aggravate or initiate their pain.

Details of how cognitive therapists do this are outside the scope of this book. Indeed, they would require another book of the same size to explain. Suffice it to say here that if you have chronic pain, it would do you no harm to ask whether your local Pain Clinic employs cognitive-behavioural therapy techniques (the two are often combined). If it does, try to get on their course.

Psychophysiology

Cognitive therapy is a form of 'mind over matter' in that the mind has transcended or banished the physical feeling of pain. It is closely linked with what is perhaps another example of mind over matter: the psychophysiological approach to pain.

Psychophysiology is based on the fact that how we think, and our emotions, can alter physiological reactions in the body. Take one example. Boxers in a ring are 'fired up' for their fight. Their bloodstream is full of adrenaline. This causes the heart to race, their physical and mental reactions to speed up, and their digestive system to shut down, as the primitive urge to fight or flee is stimulated. In this state they can tolerate far harder punches than if someone caught them unawares outside the ring. Their pain threshold is much higher than normal during the fight. Otherwise, how could boxers ever climb into the ring?

Psychophysiological approaches to pain aim to harness this ability to alter the perception of pain, without, of course, the need to stoke up the aggression needed by the boxer. There are five main ways in which people are taught to control their pain:

- control of breathing;
- relaxation;
- self-hypnosis;
- biofeedback;
- meditation.

Not all of these techniques are suitable for everyone, but you may find one that suits you. I have already covered relaxation in Chapter 10. Breath control can be practised by anyone. When we are in pain, we breathe faster and less deeply: if this continues, we pitch into a panic reaction. Understanding how to control and slow down our breathing is critical: by doing so, we slow down all our heightened bodily activities, and our pain perception is lessened. Learning breathing control takes time and a good teacher. Most Pain Clinics teach it, but if you need more help, you could do no better than an elementary yoga class. Most yoga teachers will help with meditation, too.

Self-hypnosis sounds a bit off-beat, but it is simply a technique to help you relax and turn off your brain's reception of pain. Odette Churchill's 'cinema screen' was a form of it. In biofeedback, you are taught to consciously 'think down' your pain. It has also been used to control other aspects of your physiology, such as high blood pressure. People with high blood pressure have been taught to tell themselves, inwardly, to reduce their pressure and to imagine the reading going down in their mind's eye. It has been reported to work, although modern blood pressure-lowering drugs are much more effective. 'Thinking down' one's pain is probably marginally effective, too.

All these techniques will be explained to you either by your GP or by the Pain Clinic staff. Such methods do need a lot of work and time, so do not expect quick results. Sadly, too, do not hold out your hopes that they will always work, or that when they do work they will banish the pain completely. Sometimes the best you can hope for is that they make unbearable pain bearable.

13

Chronic back pain – recovering your mobility

With chronic back pain comes limited movement, and often disability enough to cause people to become invalids and to lose their jobs. Recognition of this has led some researchers to try a completely different approach to managing chronic back pain. Instead of focusing on the pain, they focus on correcting the disability, regardless of the pain. They reason that pain is subjective, and cannot be measured. Loss of a muscle function is objective and can be measured. It can also be more important than the pain, as it may well be the main reason for the loss of a job and the diminution of the person's quality of life.

This technique is called 'functional restoration'. Pioneered by Mayer and Gatchel (Mayer and Gatchel, 1988), it depends on the premise that if you improve the way the body functions mechanically, the pain lessens anyway. Simply lessening the pain without improving function is not helpful, because the patient will still not be able to go back to work or return to a normal social and family life.

In a functional restoration laboratory, machines are used to measure the ability of muscles to move through their intended range, their strength, their endurance of exercise, and their capacity to use oxygen during tasks that imitate the movements they make at work. The subjects (this word is more appropriate than 'patients', as the work is still controversial) are then asked to undergo a month-long course of intense exercise that increases daily, and are measured again. Their pain is not taken into account: everything depends on their ability to improve their exercise capacity, to strengthen their muscles, and then to get back to their usual place in society. The team helping each person includes a doctor (to make sure that the person is in no danger), physiotherapists (to oversee their exercises) and occupational therapists (to help to rehabilitate them and eventually get them back to work).

The first results of functional restoration were brilliant, with more than 80 per cent of the subjects successfully returning to work. However, they were all American, and the trials could be criticized for lack of good control subjects as comparison. When Norwegian doctors tried to repeat their success, the results were disappointing.

They subjected 66 people who had been off work (mainly labourers) for more than a year to four weeks of exercises, group sessions, psychiatric assessments and job advice. Less than a third had returned to work within six months, and after a further year, fewer than a quarter were still in work.

Canadian and Finnish studies have followed. They showed that there was some improvement in muscle function after around three months, but it did not last for a whole year. They mirrored the Norwegian, rather than the American, results. So the jury is still out on functional restoration. Why the American results should differ so much from the others may depend on different attitudes and pressures to return to work, rather than the effect on pain.

Frankly, if the chapters on chronic pain have confused you, you are not alone. Doctors are still unsure of the best way to treat chronic low back pain. There are plenty of guidelines set by the authorities in many countries for doctors to follow, to help people with acute low back pain. These were summarized in Chapter 7. There are no such guidelines, as yet, for chronic back pain. However, while we wait for much-needed further research into better treatments for chronic back pain, here are a few thoughts on how people with it can best be treated today:

- Most people need regular analgesic drugs such as aspirin, or non-steroidal anti-inflammatory drugs (NSAIDs) such as ibuprofen, indomethacin or naproxen. They may also need antidepressants to control pain further and raise mood. Stronger drugs, such as the morphine-like opioids, should be avoided as they cause dependence and addiction, and their effect on pain is soon lost unless the dose is raised in fairly large and rapid steps. If stronger drugs than NSAIDs must be used, because the pain is so severe, then it should only be for a maximum of a week to ten days.

- Active physical therapy is a must. This means an exercise programme to get the muscles and joints working again, regardless of the pain. The aim is to become fitter generally, stronger, better co-ordinated, more supple, more mobile and to have a better posture. These active exercises are far more important than 'passive' treatments such as massage and passive physiotherapy. Occupational therapy – being given something constructive to do while you are recovering – can help towards returning to work and becoming independent again. It also bolsters confidence that you are becoming less of an invalid.

- Getting back to work and to a normal social life is also a must. Once people with chronic back pain are off work for more than six months it is very difficult to return to work. That can destroy not just a career, but a marriage and other family relationships. If you can't do what you used to do, then you need a full professional assessment of what you can do, and how it can fit with a new career. That means a team to assess how bad your pain is now and how it will progress, and an assessment of your intended job and how you will be able to cope with it physically and mentally.

- Your mental attitude matters. So if you are down and dispirited, you need psychological support. A person in pain can be helped by experts in its mental management, as well as its physical relief. You may need to attend sessions with professionals who have psychological and psychiatric backgrounds, either as an individual appointment or within a group.

- Finally, the pain may be so persistent that you may need injections to block the nerve carrying the pain message or into 'trigger points'. They can help initially, but only at the start of your rehabilitation programme. Their aim is to ease the pain so that you can become more mobile. They are not intended to be repeated just to ease pain. If the pain remains intolerable after all this, you may be assessed for surgery. That sounds hopeful, but it isn't. Very few people with chronic back pain are suitable for surgery. There is no spinal problem that an operation can cure. The vast majority of people with back pain who are sent to specialist surgeons (orthopaedic or neurosurgeons) leave the consultation disappointed because they are told there is no operation that can help them. The next chapter explains why.

14

Seeing a specialist – is your journey really necessary?

Around 9 per cent of all British adults, four million people, consult their family doctors for back pain each year (McCormick and colleagues, 1995). One in ten of these consultations is in the patient's home because the pain is so severe. The diagnoses made by the GPs range from sprains in younger adults to disc problems in middle age and osteoarthritis in the elderly. Whether these are true diagnoses or are inaccurate surmises based on unsubstantiated medical beliefs about pain and age is difficult to know.

Most of the people seen by GPs for back pain are reassured, advised to rest (perhaps unwisely), and given painkilling drugs. Those whose pain persists for a few months are X-rayed, and about one in five of them are referred to a hospital. In the meantime they may be seen by a physiotherapist, an osteopath or chiropractor.

Depending on the GP's initial diagnosis, the person with back pain will normally be referred to one of four specialists. The most common referral is to an orthopaedic surgeon. The others are a rheumatologist (a physician specializing in inflammatory disease), a Pain Clinic physician or a neurosurgeon. A small number of men, in whom prostate trouble is suspected, will see a genito-urinary surgeon.

Apart from this last small group, in whom the consultation is urgent because cancer may be suspected, most people with back pain can expect a long wait before they see their appropriate consultant. Even in hospitals, such as the Hope Hospital in South Manchester, with a research interest in back pain, only 29 per cent of patients referred to the orthopaedic department were seen within four months of their visit to their GP (South Manchester Study, 1994). By this time their back pain was severe, with more than 90 per cent of them having had it for at least three months over the previous year. Only 10 per cent of them were doing full-time work, and more than 60 per cent were not working because of their disability.

Even more ominous for GPs like myself, more than a third of this group had already been sent to other specialists, who had been unable to give them adequate help. The Hope Hospital in South

Manchester was no more successful than their previous consultations had been. Three months after their visit to the hospital, more than 90 per cent still had their backache. Understandably, 48 per cent of them were disappointed by their visit.

Why are we so inefficient in handling our patients with back pain? It all hinges on the initial diagnosis of the cause of acute back pain. Remember that 95 per cent of all back pain is not due to disease but to a functional disturbance, or misuse of the back muscles. The pain is not caused by anything wrong with any structure in the back, so no amount of investigations or surgical treatment will put it right. GPs, though, faced with patients who keep returning because their pain is not cured, feel they must make sure that they have not overlooked something that a specialist can deal with.

Hence the massive numbers of visitors to orthopaedic, neurosurgical and rheumatological clinics. When one consultant cannot find a cause and cure, the reasoning goes that perhaps another can. It may be cynical, but GPs may be forgiven for thinking that while the patient is waiting to see yet another consultant, they have some respite from having to deal with the problem themselves.

This only postpones the ultimate responsibility for the family doctor. Many backache sufferers, having pinned their hopes on their visit to the consultant, find them dashed when they are told that there is no suitable surgery or – in the case of the rheumatologist – no other medical treatment for their pain. They are back to square one, often having had several back X-rays and maybe even CAT (computer-assisted tomography) or an MRI (magnetic resonance imaging) scan. They are back in the hands of their GPs, still with their pain, but this time with all other options exhausted. They are faced with having to manage their back pain themselves.

You think this may be exaggerated, that I am looking on the black side? Then consider the report of the Clinical Standards Advisory Group (CSAG) in 1994 on the management of back pain. I take them from Professor Waddell's book, *The Back Pain Revolution*. At the time of writing, the CSAG figures are eight years or so out of date, so they may even be underestimating the problem.

CSAG estimates that in any one year, sixteen million people have back pain, and around four to six million consult their GPs about their pain. Some 1,600,000 are referred to hospital outpatient clinics for their back pain; and 100,000 are admitted to hospital because of back pain. Some 24,000 are operated on – that is, they have surgery to discs or have vertebrae fused.

A quick calculation of these figures shows that only one in around seventy people with back pain needs surgery to relieve it. It also means that there are hundreds of thousands of people on the hospital referral treadmill who need not be there, who will not be helped even by the most prestigious and conscientious consultant. The consultants know this, and so do the GPs. Now you know it, too.

Of course, there are people who really need to be sent to hospital. They are the people mentioned on pages 4–5 with the 'red flags' of symptoms that need urgent attention. They are the people whose bulging discs are causing concern because their muscles are weakened, their limbs are numb and beset with pins and needles, and they are having problems with their bladder and bowels. Their GPs are trained to spot them, and to admit them to hospital as urgent or emergency cases. The figures show that they are a very small proportion of all people with back pain – probably between 1 and 2 per cent.

For the other 98 per cent, perhaps one answer would be to reorganize the consultant services. There should be more specialist Pain Clinics, in which anaesthetists and other people interested in dealing with pain get together not just to treat the pain, but to reorganize the back-pain sufferer's whole life. In such clinics, drugs to ease pain would only be a small part of the treatment, and complex investigations involving scans would be very firmly in the distant background. This would allow the orthopaedic surgeons, the neurosurgeons and rheumatologists to get on with investigating the people they really need to see. It would be a huge relief for all of them, and, more important, for everyone with back pain.

15

When the specialist is necessary

If you are in the small minority of back-pain sufferers who really need to see a specialist, how do you know? Perhaps the best way to explain is to follow the recommended 'triage' of any person coming to the doctor with low back pain. The doctor has to answer a series of questions about the patient, the answers to which lead on to the action to be taken and to the next question. The questions go as follows:

1 Is the pain due to a problem in the back or elsewhere? If it is elsewhere, as in the abdomen, kidneys, gallbladder, circulation or linked to a general disease, then the illness has to be identified and managed appropriately, either by the GP or by a hospital referral to the corresponding specialist. If it is primarily a back problem, then go to question 2.

2 Is there a difficulty in passing urine, a problem with walking and or balance, and numbness around the anus and perineum? If there is, then the person needs emergency admission to a spinal surgery unit, to take the pressure off the lower spinal cord. If none of these problems are present, then go to question 3.

3 Has the patient got serious spinal disease? Among the symptoms that would suggest this are: a patient younger than 20 or older than 55, with pain not related to position or activity, in the chest as well as the back, who is obviously unwell, losing weight, with other symptoms relating to nerve damage or irritation, with an obvious deformity of the back, or has HIV, a known cancer, or is on long-term steroids. Any of these require urgent referral to the appropriate specialist. If none of these conditions are present, then go to question 4.

4 Is there a nerve root problem? Signs are a pain in one leg that is worse than the pain in the back, that goes as far as the foot and toes, with numbness, weakness and pins and needles in the same area as the pain. The pain can be reproduced by raising the leg straight up while the patient is lying on the back. If the answer is yes, then go to question 5. If the answer is no, go to question 7.

5 Is there, along with the nerve root problem, severe weakness in

the leg that is worsening rapidly? If yes, the patient must be sent urgently into hospital. If no, the GP should follow up the patient at home for around four weeks, initiating the usual exercise and pain relief therapy mentioned in Chapter 7. On the follow-up meeting, go to question 6.

6 After one month of treatment, is the pain settling? If no, then the patient should be sent to the local hospital specialist who deals with spinal nerve root problems. He may be an orthopaedic surgeon or a spinal neurosurgeon. If yes, then home care by the GP can continue, and the patient can return to work.

7 The patient has simple backache, and does not need to go to hospital. Care can be undertaken by the GP team, and there is no need to stay off work.

Again it must be emphasized that the vast majority of people with backache get to question 7. Only a small minority have to be treated by a specialist team. On the whole, specialists in Britain are more reluctant to operate on backs than those in the United States. Amazingly, in the United States, spinal surgery is the third most common operation, after female sterilization and caesarian section. Most of the operations are fusions of two vertebrae, either in the neck or lower back, to relieve nerve root pressure.

In Britain, spinal surgery is well down the list of common operations. Disc operations (removing bulging areas of disc) are much more common than fusions in the United Kingdom. In 1990, the last year I can find statistics for, there were 12,000 lumbar disc operations and only 1,100 fusions. There were only 857 operations for spinal deformities. Numbers of operations have probably risen since then, but not dramatically: the pattern of surgery is probably still the same. What is difficult to find out is how successful the surgery is in eliminating the pain. My suspicion is that in Britain, where the specialists are much less likely to operate, people who are operated upon are those who need surgery the most, not just to ease their pain, but to prevent incontinence from damage to the nerves controlling the bladder and bowel. In Britain, where spinal surgery is always the last resort, the results may well be better in terms of easing pain than in countries where it is used more readily.

Types of surgery to the spine

In researching this book, I was intrigued by an old Consumers'

Association publication, *Avoiding Back Trouble*, published in 1975. It starts its section on surgery with the following: 'No guarantee is ever given beforehand by a surgeon that a spinal operation will be a success. However, the majority are successful – otherwise surgeons would not continue doing them.'

I'd like to think that was true, but it is difficult to find hard evidence to prove or disprove that optimistic piece of logic. The history of surgery is littered with operations that did not do much good, but were continued for years before they were discarded. I hope the same is not true for spinal surgery, but every GP has been faced with people who still have their back pain after having had radical surgery to their backs.

So no one should contemplate back surgery lightly. To be fair to the modern British spinal surgeons, none of them advise operating unless they are very sure that it is essential for that particular patient. It is never a question of routine. Each person has a unique back problem, and the pre-surgery assessment must encompass all of its details.

If surgery is being considered, your surgeon will explain beforehand exactly why it is needed, and what is being done. You will be asked to give consent to it, in the full knowledge of its chances of success and of its possible complications. You will also be told beforehand how you will feel afterwards, and how you will have to co-operate with the recovery room and rehabilitation staff in the days and weeks that follow.

There are three classical reasons for operating on spines. The first is to relieve the pressure on nerve roots in the gaps between vertebrae. The most common cause of this pressure is a bulging disc, and the aim is to remove the bulge. This is often called 'discectomy' even though the whole disc may not be removed. Another cause is a projecting piece of vertebral bone, which will need 'nibbling away'.

The second type of operation, 'fusion', is done to make a 'loose' joint between vertebrae more stable. It is done to make solid, or fuse together, the joints between two or even three adjacent vertebrae so that there is no movement between them. The aim is to ensure that the gap between the vertebrae, through which nerves pass, is always wide enough not to 'nip' the nerve, and cannot be narrowed by bending the back in any direction. In spinal fusion, the surgeon forms a 'bridge' between the target joints with a piece of the patient's own bone (usually from just behind the upper rim of the pelvis). Screws, clips, plates and springs may be used to keep it in place until the bone grafts on to the vertebrae naturally. In the United States the operation is sometimes performed using artificial material (a 'prosthesis') to bridge the gap, but results so far do not suggest that this is more effective than using bone.

Sometimes the preferred operation is to remove the 'roof' of a vertebra (its back surface when you are standing), which widens the space in which the spinal cord lies, thereby relieving pressure on it. This is laminectomy. Often a small laminectomy is done to get access to a bulging disc, so that many spinal operations that are not strictly laminectomies are given that label. A laminectomy may also be done during a fusion operation to make it easier to apply the bone graft.

In a few people, the pressure on nerve roots does not come from discs but from 'spicules' of bones jutting towards the spinal cord and nerves from the small side joints of the vertebrae. These joints are called facet joints, so the operation is called 'facetectomy'. If the surgeon has to do a wide facetectomy, then it is usually combined with a spinal fusion. In yet others, their pain arises from pressure below the lumbar spine, inside the spinal canal at the level of the pelvis. This is 'cauda equina' pressure, and must be relieved if incontinence and weakness and permanent numbness of the legs are to be avoided. The surgeon will achieve this by opening up the dura mater, the tough protective covering around the spinal cord.

You would think that with all the detail that surgeons can gather, using MRI scans, about your spine before they embark on surgery, you might be told what operation you are going to have in advance. That isn't the case. You may be told that the likely operation will be a discectomy, but find afterwards that you have had a full spinal fusion. This isn't the surgeon's fault: it is often impossible to tell exactly what is needed until the operation starts and the true extent of the problem is laid bare. You will have to accept that the surgeon has discretion on what to do after he has you on the surgical table.

You would also think that after what seems to you fairly major surgery that you will have to rest for a few weeks afterwards. That isn't the case either. Gone are the days, thankfully, when people had to lie on their backs for months after spinal surgery. Now they are up and about in a few days, obviously in the careful hands of the nurses and physiotherapists, so that they can become mobile again as quickly as possible. There will be positions to avoid, such as curling up in bed, sitting in low chairs with the legs out straight, or bending over. But on the whole, you will be surprised at how much freedom you will have to move around, and by the vigorous exercises you will be asked to do, quite soon after surgery. The timing and the extent of your rehabilitation programme will depend on what you have had done and your physical fitness and abilities. If you are going to have surgery, make sure that you know what lies ahead for you: your surgical and physiotherapy teams will be happy to discuss it with you in detail.

After the immediate recovery period, it is you who will determine how fast you will return to normal life and work. The harder you work at it the sooner you will be back to normal. Your doctor and physiotherapist can only advise you: it is your job to take that advice.

Occupational therapy

As you are recovering, you will meet your occupational therapist. In Britain, occupational therapists are state registered and have completed a three-year training. They assess the physical abilities of their clients and advise them on what they can and cannot do physically. They also help people make the most of the abilities they have and help them back into work that they can perform. You may meet the occupational therapist in a workshop or in a gymnasium: the therapist will plan a programme for you that will probably include both.

When the time comes for you to go back to work, the occupational therapist will assess your intended job, and what it involves in physical workload. This does not just mean whether you are lifting heavy weights in an awkward way – most reasonable employers ensure that people do not do that today. It may mean, however, an analysis of how many hours you sit or stand in one position, and whether the seat or the standing position can be improved so that you no longer put stress on your back. The occupational therapist may even wish to watch you at work, to make sure that you are using the right muscles in the right way, and not slipping back into the habits that gave you the back pain to begin with.

Occupational therapy isn't just about men and women at work. It is also about them in the home, too. Hospital occupational therapy departments contain model kitchens, bathrooms and bedrooms, to put men and women through their routines in the home. Tasks done in a manner likely to initiate back pain again are noted and you are shown how to change things to minimize the risk. You may be asked to repeat back-saving tasks over and over again, so that they are 'imprinted' on you when you go home. Your doctor can arrange for occupational therapists working in the district, and employed by the local authority, to visit your home. They will ensure that it is 'back friendly' and will recommend ways in which things can be changed to save your back. If the changes are expensive and you are entitled to financial relief, the social services department should have funds to help pay for them.

Many of the changes you can make yourself, fairly easily. Simply changing the height of a working surface, a sink, or a shelf to stop you stooping or leaning forward or stretching upwards for hours at a time, may be all that you need to do. Choosing a different chair at work and in the home, preferably with a high back on which you can rest your head, can make a big difference. Many companies link the type of chair you sit in with your status within the company. They would do far better if they made sure that everyone who sits for any length of time at their job had a very comfortable chair that supported their whole back and head.

Using a desk surface at an angle, like a draughtsman's board, rather than flat, can make a lot of difference to your posture at work. The position you take at a computer monitor is vital. It is far better to work looking down at a screen, rather than up at it. Constantly looking up at a screen arches the neck backwards and tenses all the muscles of the spine. Looking down at the screen relaxes the neck and the back muscles follow.

To summarize, take advice from your occupational therapist on how you can arrange your work and daily living to your advantage, and also from your physiotherapist on how much you can exercise and how best to move your limbs and torso, and you will not go far wrong.

Sex

One aspect of back pain that few books touch upon is sex. Back pain can ruin your sex life. It exhausts you, so that you don't feel like sex, and that is distressing – and in the long run very destructive for you and your partner. Even when you do feel like making love, it can bring on an attack of back pain, and that can be extremely frustrating for both of you.

Yet plenty of couples have found their own solutions. One is to take a painkilling tablet that you know is effective for you about an hour before you plan to have sex. Then its effects will be at their height during most of your love-making. If it is the actual movements that bring on the pain, then take as passive a role as is still satisfying for you. Or find an active role, in a different position, that doesn't bring on the pain. It is often a matter of trial and error, but it can be a lot of fun discovering what works for you, and you can laugh together later about what doesn't. There are plenty of books on sexual techniques that you can follow, if you have a mind to. Most couples find their own solutions without them. The overriding message throughout this book is that exercise is more effective than rest. Sex is an exercise, too.

16
Getting active – a few details

We all spend time every day on our appearance. Men shave, women put on make-up, both spend time on their hair, and try to keep clean, fresh and presentable. But we do little to keep our backs in good shape. Most of us assume that our daily work, whether at the office or factory or in the house, keeps us physically active enough without the need to do extra exercise.

It is true that we don't really need to do specific back exercises to keep supple and fit. All we need to do is to set aside enough time each day to perform normal activities like walking, cycling or swimming. Or even ballroom dancing if you prefer. Yet few of us actually do this. And driving or sitting all day leaves many of us with stiff and painful backs.

One restriction to good back health is our clothing. Tight skirts and belted trousers restrict the range of movements we can make. For example, they stop you bending your knees enough to lift objects. Your limbs and back need to be put through their full range of movements regularly. So if you know that you need to be flexible through the day, dress accordingly. Fashion doesn't need to take precedent over comfort at work.

Being overweight is a drawback. It makes it even more difficult to move fully, and the extra weight can accelerate the degenerative changes that happen to us all as we age, especially in weight-bearing joints such as in the spine, the hips, knees and ankles. So, even though there is no proof from reliable trials that losing weight will directly ease your back pain (see page 25), it is always helpful for your general health to lose the extra pounds. And by now you will have guessed that the experts' advice on how to do that is to exercise more!

If you decide on walking for your exercise, walk with your spine upright and head held high. Don't stoop or shuffle. If you are carrying anything, have it on your back so that its weight is central over your spine, and not on one side. A rucksack-type bag is preferable to a shoulder bag. If you choose cycling, make sure your bike is one with upright handlebars so that your back is straight, rather than racing-type ones that cause you to hunch your back and shoulders. When you are swimming, alternate your strokes: I enjoy a rotation of three lengths, one crawl, one breaststroke and one backstroke. That way you exercise all the muscles, and make use of all the muscles around the spine in turn.

Back exercises

As for exercises specifically to loosen up your back, I'm not really a fan of them. As I have written elsewhere in this book, there is little evidence that they help any more than just getting on with normal activities like walking or swimming. But I have added a few of them here for completeness. If you are stiff, as well as in pain, and you haven't the time or inclination (or right weather!) to go out for a walk, these exercises can loosen you up, which usually relieves the pain.

The exercises start from different positions – lying face up (supine), face down (prone), on one side, standing, and sitting. You do not have to do them all in any one day. Chose a set of exercises that you feel like doing at the time, and mix and match a little. If you haven't exercised for a time, start with the easiest and progress a bit further as you feel more supple, day by day.

Supine exercises

Lying on your back, raise a knee up to a right angle from the hip, so that the shin is horizontal, then in a series of small rhythmic movements bend it further back and up until the front of the thigh is close to your tummy and chest. Repeat with the other leg. Relax for a minute, then bend up one knee, keeping the foot on the floor. Swing the knee from one side to the other as far as it will go without discomfort for a few minutes. Repeat with the other knee. Relax again. Now bend both knees up with the feet still on the floor. Keeping the shoulders and buttocks touching the floor, raise and lower the small of your back, so that it is first arched, then flattened. Again, with both knees raised and feet on the floor, this time raise the buttocks off the floor and lower them again, several times. Relax again.

Now, still supine, bend your knees again leaving your feet under the edge of a wardrobe or a mattress or low chair. Stretching your hand forwards, lift your shoulders to curl up your back as far forward as you can. This should be a smooth, gentle process, not a jerky one. Relax back. Repeat several times and relax again. Once you have done this a few times you should be able to sit upright from the supine position. Next, still supine, bend one knee until the thigh is vertical. Now, with the thigh in this position, straighten the leg until the whole leg is pointing at the ceiling. Put your arms out to the side to stabilize yourself, then bend the straight leg over first to one side, then to the other. Do the same with the other leg, and relax. Repeat several times and relax again.

Prone exercises

Lying on your front, you may have to put a thin pillow under your abdomen if your back is painful. Now bend your knees so that the lower legs are vertical. Drop your heels down towards your buttocks and raise them again, one leg at a time. Relax. Now bend one knee up again, and drop it outwardly and back to the vertical, to each side alternately. Do the same with the other leg and relax. Then bend both knees to the vertical, and lift each thigh up and down, as far as you can, alternately. Now do the same with both thighs at the same time. Relax again, and after about a minute, still prone, raise each leg, first alternately, then together, with knees straight, as far as you can. Now, with either someone to hold your feet down, or with them tucked under the edge of a chair or other similar furniture, slowly raise and lower your head and shoulders. Try to increase gradually the height by which you raise them.

Standing exercises

Stand upright with your back straight. Put your hands straight out in front of you on a chair or other piece of furniture at an appropriate height. Now bend and straighten your knees while keeping your back straight. Take it gently at first, and gradually increase the bend. Stand still for a moment, then bend each knee upwards, gradually pulling them nearer to your chest.

Now take your hands off the chair. Place them on the front of your thighs and slide them down towards the knees, bending your head down as you do so. Allow your back to curl forward as you do this. Straighten and bend again, this time going a little further down your legs. Eventually you will be able to touch your feet – or at least get much closer to them than before. However, ask your doctor beforehand if this exercise is correct for you. For some people with disc problems it may not be. Stand relaxed for a minute, then raise one thigh until it is horizontal, and keep it there as you straighten and bend the knee several times. Do the same for the other leg. Stand for a minute, then bend your spine to one side and then the other, sliding the appropriate hand down the side as you do so.

Now return to the chair, and swing each leg in turn back and forwards, then to the side and back in again. Repeat several times before resting again. Now leave the chair, and stand with your feet wide apart. Turn your body and feet towards one side and make a lunging movement forward, so that the front leg is bent and the back leg straight. Stand straight again, turn to the other direction, and repeat the exercise.

Sitting exercises

Now sit on the chair (it should have a straight back and no arms), with feet on the floor and hips and knees at right angles. With your knees still bent, raise them alternately up to your chest. Then relax. Still sitting, straighten each knee, and use your thigh muscles to hold them horizontally for twenty or so seconds. Finally, sit with your knees apart and your hands on your knees. Bend your body forward while keeping your head straight, so that your shoulders drop between your knees. Raise your body again, and repeat several times.

To finish the exercise you can 'hang' from your fingers from the top of a door or a convenient beam. You don't have to have your feet off the floor, just allow yourself to sag with your feet forward and your knees straight. After that, lie flat, supine, for a few minutes before rolling to one side and getting up, keeping your back straight as you do so. You may well be surprised by how good – and how tall – you feel after all these simple exercises.

17
Closing thoughts

Any author will admit that books never turn out to be quite what was planned, and that goes for factual books like this one, just as much as for fiction. I was struck, as I was doing the background research, by the very comprehensive literature and very detailed scientific trials that showed time and again that the vast majority of cases of back pain, no matter how crippling they seemed, were not due to spinal disease. They were simple muscular pains that could be managed well by their 'owners' themselves.

Yet there is a huge medical and paramedical industry that has grown up around back pain. GPs like myself spend many hours sending back-pain sufferers into the treadmill of orthopaedic and neurosurgical clinics, only to receive most of them back no better. That is largely because the hospital specialists, having found nothing wrong that they can put right with surgery, have no answer for their pain. Of course, there are a few exceptions to this rule: I have often quoted Professor Waddell throughout this book. If only there were a lot more like him.

I don't blame the orthopaedic or neurosurgical specialists. They are there to do their job, which is to correct serious diseases of the spine, and not to sift through the many people with simple back problems who are sent to them by GPs who do not know what to do with them. The specialists must be just as frustrated with this as we GPs are – and as are the patients themselves.

Proof of this comes from two sources. Professor Waddell compares the treatment of back pain by hospital specialists in the United States and the United Kingdom. One person in five sent to an orthopaedic surgeon or neurosurgeon in the United States for simple back pain is eventually operated upon. The corresponding figure for Britain is under 3 per cent. Professor Waddell states that American medical care for back pain is 'too fragmented, too specialized, too invasive and too expensive'. He describes the British NHS care for back pain as 'more cohesive, but under-funded, too little and too late'. He continues, 'Yet despite the very different health care systems, there is little evidence that they make much difference to the social impact of back pain in the two countries.'

The same goes not just for medical specialists, but for the alternatives. Whether or not there is easy access to osteopaths and chiropractors in an area makes no difference to the back-pain workload. So these practitioners are not curing the condition, either.

I can only agree with Professor Waddell. We have been getting the treatment of back pain spectacularly wrong, and we need to put it right. Essential to this is that you, the person with the pain, should understand what is causing it, and how you can manage it yourself. It is not a medical or surgical problem. It may be a postural problem, or a problem of excessive workload, or how you spend your leisure time, or just a problem of getting your muscles right. Your lifestyle matters just as much, and probably even more, than your medication or your need for surgery. Your muscles need to be in tune, in tone, and to relax once in a while. How many of us actually understand that, then put it into practice?

I've been typing for four hours today without a break, first on a draft for an article, then on this last chapter. Because I wanted to get them right, I sat too long in the same position. I now have backache, and must get up and walk around and stretch. It's only a minor inconvenience, and at least I have the answer at my fingertips. Everybody should have the same choice, regardless of their work or position. In the final analysis, the hard work of treating backache has to come from the person with the pain. Doctors and alternative practitioners are only on the periphery, and that's where we should probably remain.

References

Barlow, W., *The Alexander Principle*. London, Arrow Books, 1986.

Battie, M. C., *et al.*, 'Smoking and lumbar intervertebral disc degeneration: an MRI study of identical twins', *Spine*, 1991, vol. 16, pp. 1015–21.

Burton, A. K., *et al.*, 'Lumbar sigittal mobility and low back symptoms in patients treated with manipulation', *Journal of Spinal Disorders*, 1990, vol. 3, pp. 262–8.

Deyo, R. A., and Bass, J. E., 'Lifestyle and low back pain: the influence of smoking and obesity', *Spine*, 1989, vol. 14, pp. 501–6.

DiGiovanna, E. L., and Schiowitz, S., *An Osteopathic Approach to Diagnosis and Treatment*. Lippincott, 1991.

Fogg, A. J. B., and Taylor, A. E., 'The usefulness of the shuttle walk test in a population of low back pain patients', presented to the International Society for the Study of the Lumbar Spine, Singapore, 1997.

Fordyce, W. E., *Behavioural Methods for Chronic Pain*. St Louis, USA, Mosby, 1976.

Frost, H., *et al.*, 'Randomised controlled trial for evaluation of fitness programme for patients with chronic low back pain', *British Medical Journal*, 1992, vol. 310, pp. 151–4.

Haldeman, S., and Rubinstein, S., 'Cauda equina syndrome in patients undergoing manipulation of the lumbar spine', *Spine*, 1992, vol. 17, pp. 1469–73.

Hall, H., *et al.*, 'The spontaneous onset of back pain', *Clinical Journal of Pain*, 1998, vol. 14, p. 2.

Hansen, F. R., *et al.*, 'Intensive dynamic back muscle exercises, conventional therapy or placebo control treatment of low back pain', *Spine*, 1993, vol. 18, pp. 98–107.

Hulshof, C., and van Zanten, B. V., 'Whole body vibration and back pain', *Internal Archives of Occupational and Environmental Health*, 1987, vol. 59, pp. 205–20.

Lindequist, S., *et al.*, 'Information and regime for low back pain', *Scandinavian Journal of Rehabilitation Medicine*, 1984, vol. 16, pp. 113–16.

REFERENCES

Lindstrom, I., *et al.*, 'Mobility, strength and fitness after a graded activity program for patients with subacute low back pain', *Spine*, 1992, vol. 17, pp. 641–52.

Linton, S. J., *et al.*, 'A controlled study of the effects of an early intervention on acute musculoskeletal pain problems', *Pain*, 1993, vol. 54, pp. 353–9.

MacFarlane, G. J., *et al.*, 'Employment and physical work activities as predictors of future low back pain', *Spine*, 1997, vol. 22, pp. 1143–9.

Manninen, P., *et al.*, 'Mental distress and disability due to low back and other musculoskeletal disorders – a ten year follow up', report to *The International Society for the Study of the Lumbar Spine*, 1995, p. 37.

Mayer, T. G., and Gatchel, R. J., *Functional Restoration for Spinal Disorders: The Sports Medicine Approach*. Philadelphia, Lea & Febiger, 1988.

McCormick, A., *et al.*, *The Fourth National Morbidity Study*. HMSO, Office of Population Censuses and Surveys Series MB5, no. 3, 1995.

Melzack, R., 'The short form McGill Pain Questionnaire', *Pain*, 1987, vol. 30, pp. 191–7.

Melzack, R., 'Gate control theory: on the evolution of pain concepts', *Pain Forum*, 1996, vol. 5, pp. 128–38.

Melzack, R., and Wall, P. D., 'Pain mechanisms: a new theory', *Science*, 1965, vol. 150, pp. 971–9.

Palmer, D. D., *The Science, Art and Philosophy of Chiropractic*. Oregon, Portland Printing House, 1910.

Pope, M. H., *et al.*, 'Biomechanics of the lumbar spine: A. Basic principles' in *The Adult Spine: Principles and Practice*, ed. J. W. Frymoyer. New York, Raven Press, 1991, pp. 1487–1501.

Roland, M., and Morris, R., 'A study of the natural history of back pain. Part 1: development of a reliable and sensitive measure of disability in low back pain', *Spine*, 1983, vol. 8, pp. 141–4.

Smith, T., *Coping Successfully with Prostate Cancer*. London, Sheldon Press, 2002.

Smith, T., and Cooper, W., *Human Potential, The Limits and Beyond*. Newton Abbot, David & Charles, 1980.

South Manchester Study, *A Report to the Clinical Standards Advisory Group of the Department of Health*. The Arthritis and Rheumatism Council, Epidemiology Research Unit, University of Manchester, 1994.

REFERENCES

Still, A. T., *Philosophy of Osteopathy*. Kirksville, USA, 1899.

The Back Book, available from the Stationery Office, St Crispins, Duke Street, Norwich NR3 1PD, or from good bookshops (ISBN 0–11–702078–8).

Troup, J. D. G., 'Drivers' back pain and its prevention', *Applied Ergonomics*, 1978, vol. 9, pp. 207–14.

van Tulder, M. W., *et al.*, *Low Back Pain in Primary Care*. Amsterdam, Institute for Research in Extramural Medicine, 1996, pp. 245–95.

Waddell, G., *The Back Pain Revolution*. London, Churchill Livingstone, 1998.

Wall, P. D., 'Comments after 30 years of the gate control theory', *Pain Forum*, 1996, vol. 5, pp. 15–22.

Index